AUTISM SPECTRUM 75 EXERCISES

Coloring with Connection
for Social Comfort &
Emotional Processing

A BRAIN TRAINING GAMES

Created by Sarah Janisse Brown The

Thinking Tree, LLC - Copyright 2023

FunSchooling.com

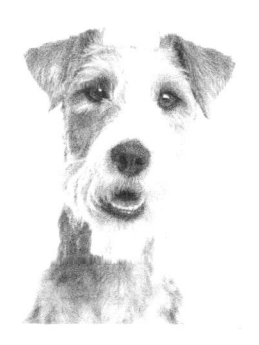

By Sarah Janisse Brown
the Creator of
Dyslexia Games Therapy
And Publisher of
Math Craft for Dyscalculia

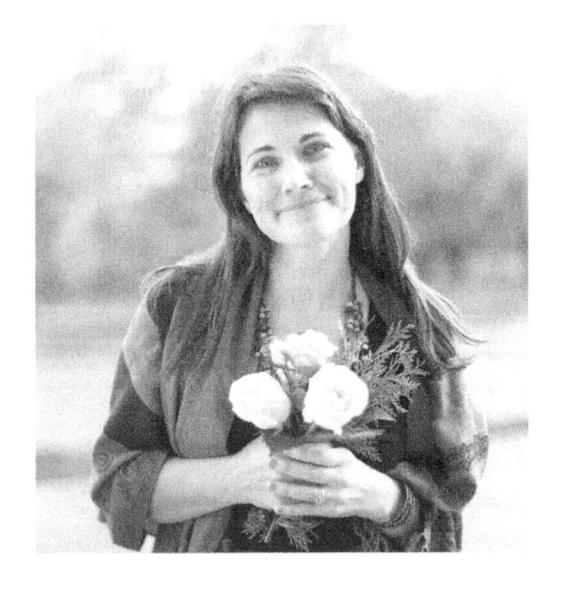

FunSchooling.com
DyslexiaGames.com

Name:

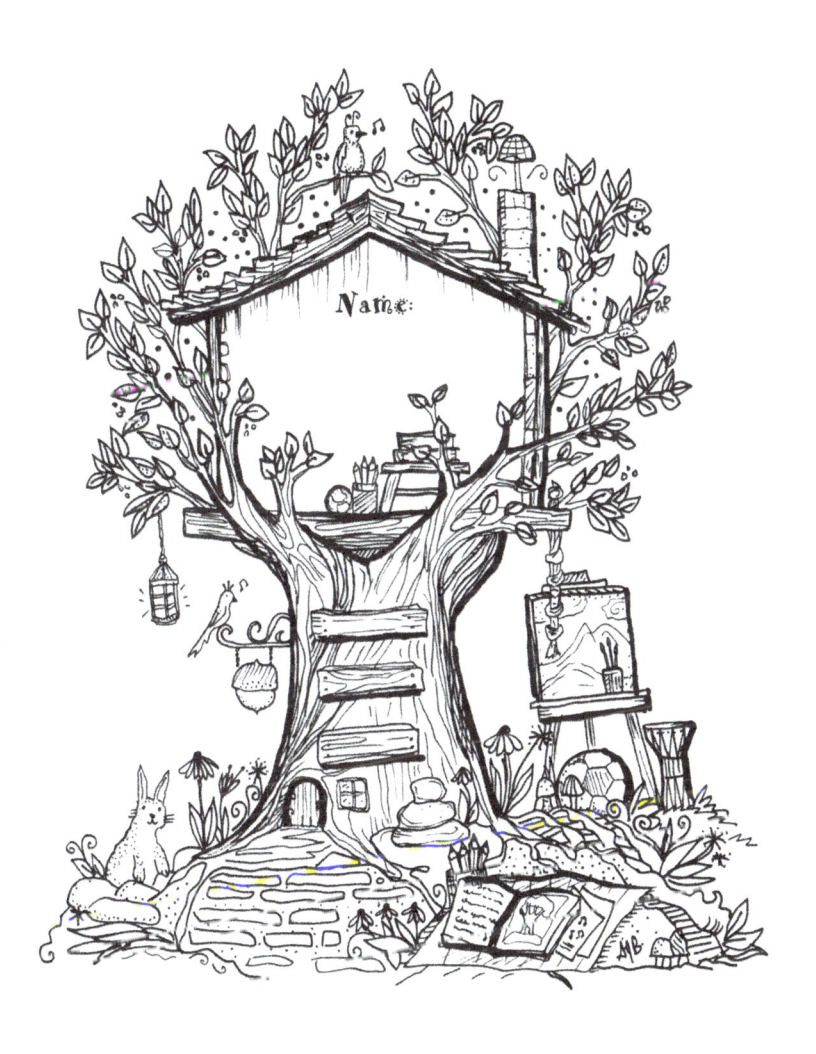

HOW TO USE THIS BOOK

This is a coloring book and activity book with fifty photos of faces, shown in grayscale, presented along with a few different thinking activities and logic games.

We present images of people of various races, and include children with disabilities and Down Syndrome. There are animal faces and human faces showing different feelings. After every five face pages there will be a "Thinking Page" where the student can freely write about their thoughts. Next is a "Draw Anything Pages" and a "Logic Page". At first it may be hard for the student to use an open ended activity page. Feel free to give the student some prompts or ask them to write about their special interest or recent experiences.

The person using the book should look at the faces and consider how each person or animal is feeling. They will color the eyes in order to become more comfortable with eye contact. If you are a parent, teacher, therapist or friend who is working with the autistic person, be open to helping with some of the activities in order to be an example. For example take turns working on each page. Talk about your feelings and the feeling of the person or animal in each picture.

The goal is for the autistic person using the book to become more interested in the faces, feelings and thoughts of others. People with autism tend to avoid looking at faces, this behavior causes them to become unaware of how people express feeling through facial expressions. When someone with autism becomes comfortable with eye contact, and becomes more interested in faces, they may begin to over come some of their social discomforts.

Many people with autism do not enjoy making eye contact. That may be because it makes them feel uncomfortable. By coloring the eyes in this book the student can become more comfortable with eyes in general. We included animals in this therapy book because it will be easier to color the pictures of the animals at first.

Parents: If you are working with a child. please feel free to allow the child to choose what page he or she wants to use first. The child can work on one face per day. Be sure to talk with your child about feelings, use a mirror and try to make the face the person or animals is making in the photo.

This concept was introduced in **2016** as a research experiment, and several children on the autism spectrum experienced improvements in social comfort and emotional understanding. The therapy is still experimental. Please leave a review to share your experience with us concerning the use of this book.

This activity book is small. We don't want it to feel intimidating or overwhelming. It's easy to take along wherever you go.

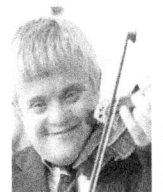

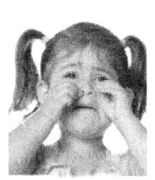

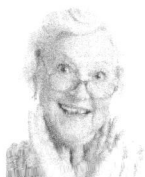

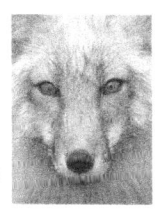

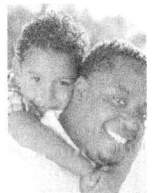

LOOK AT MY FACE!

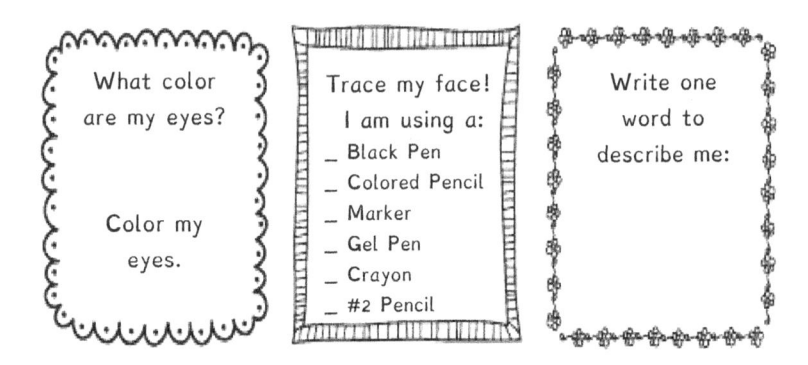

What color are my eyes?

Color my eyes.

Trace my face!
I am using a:
_ Black Pen
_ Colored Pencil
_ Marker
_ Gel Pen
_ Crayon
_ #2 Pencil

Write one word to describe me:

COLOR THE FACES THAT SHOW HOW I FEEL:

Draw me

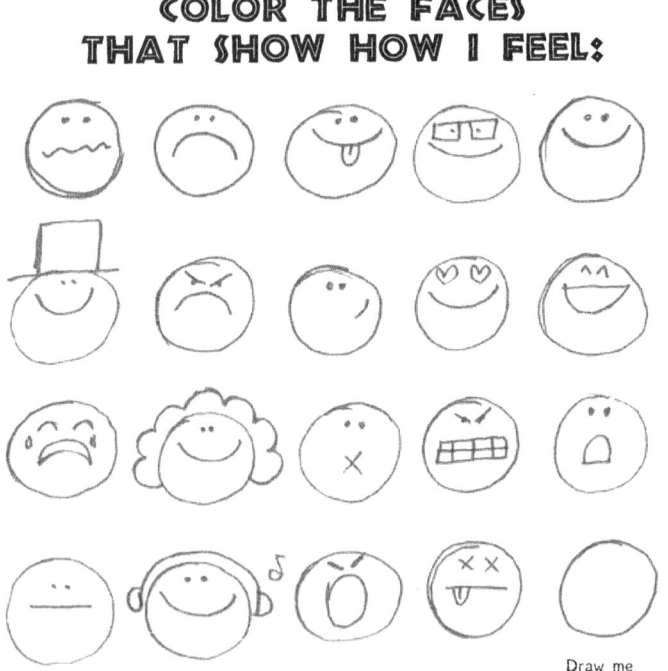

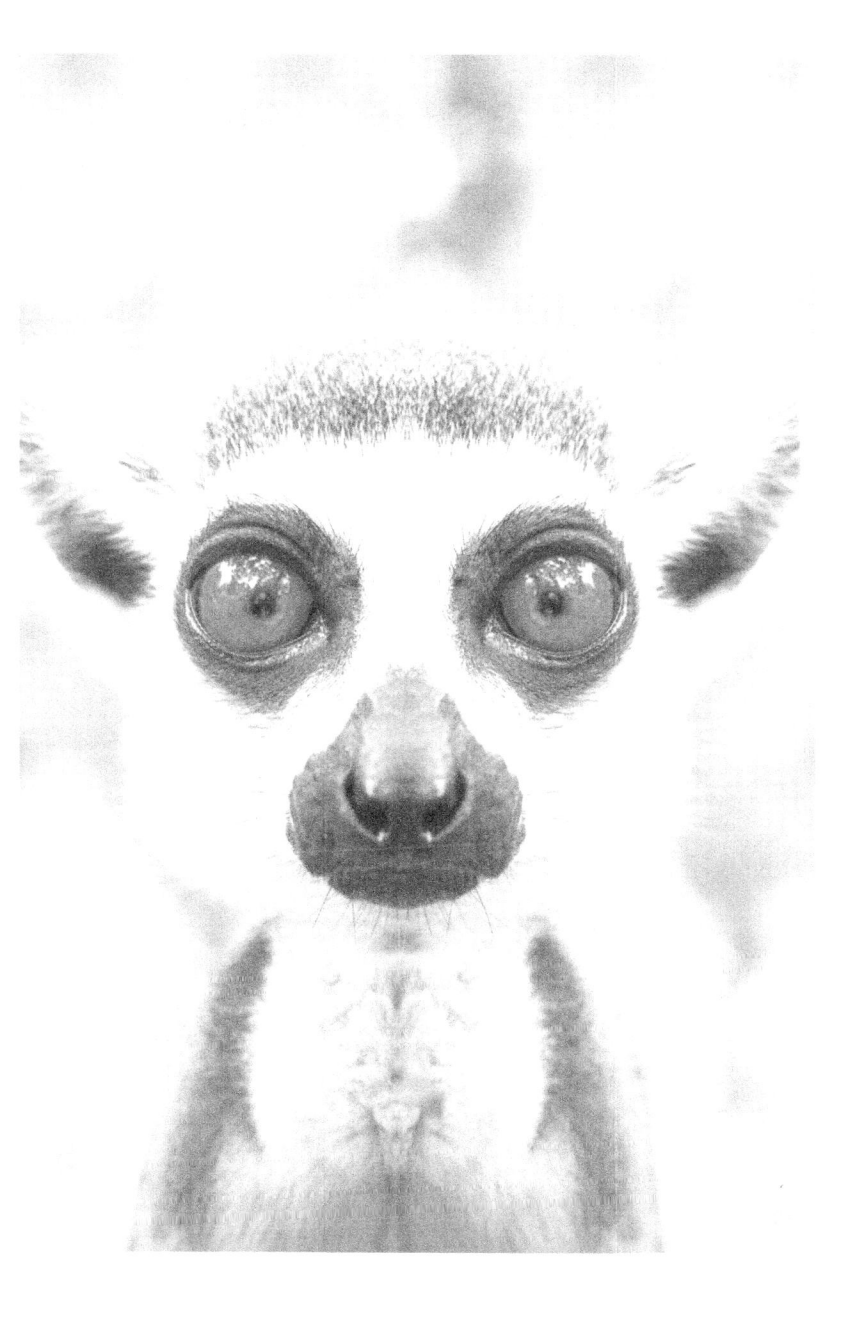

LOOK AT MY FACE!

What color are my eyes?

Color my eyes.

Trace my face!
I am using a:
_ Black Pen
_ Colored Pencil
_ Marker
_ Gel Pen
_ Crayon
_ #2 Pencil

Write one word to describe me:

COLOR THE FACES THAT SHOW HOW I FEEL:

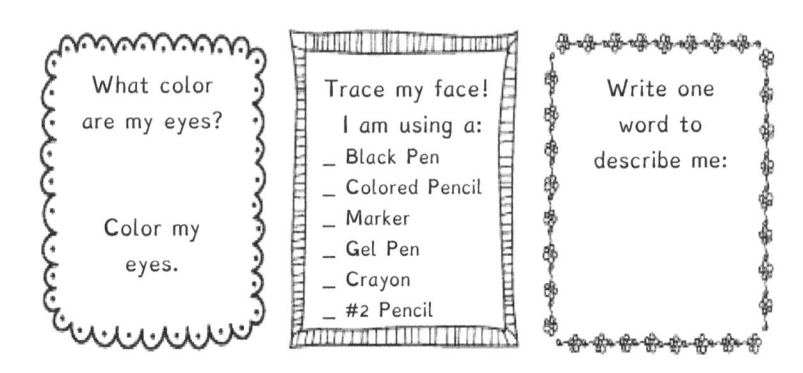

Draw me

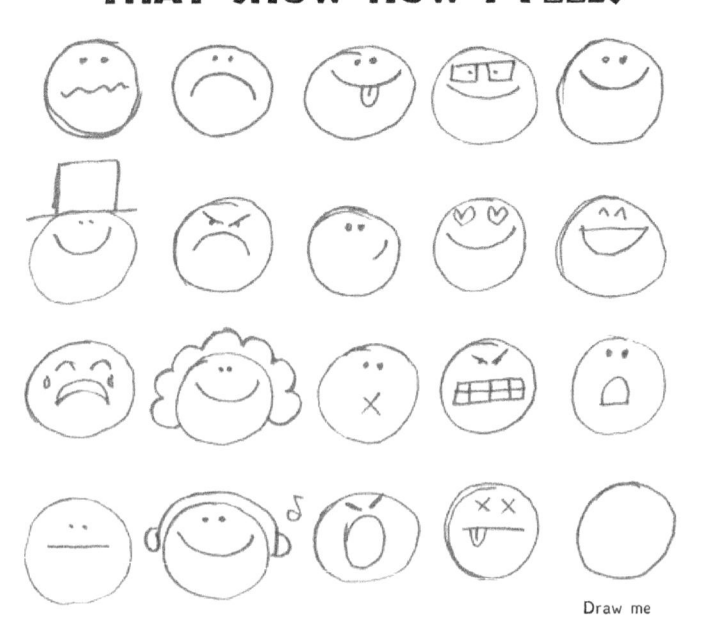

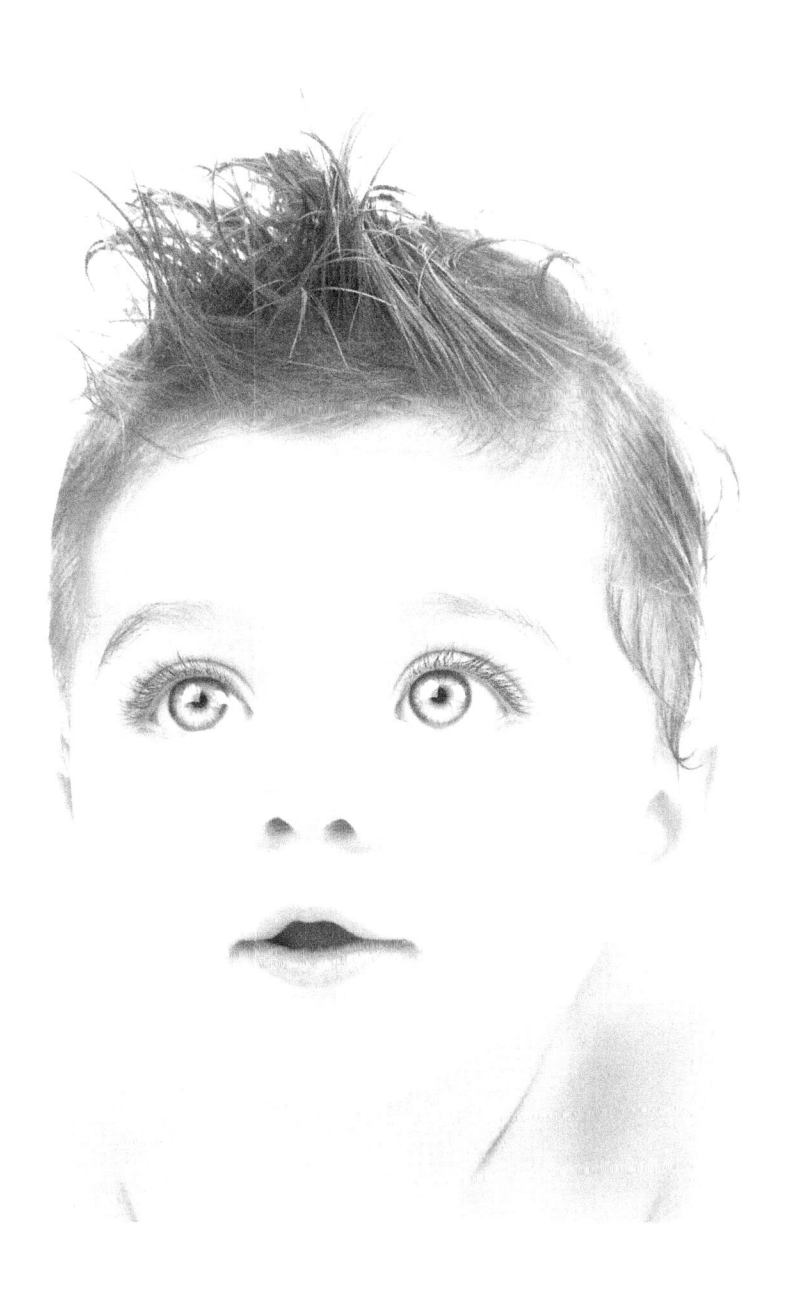

LOOK AT MY FACE!

| What color are my eyes? Color my eyes. | Trace my face! I am using a: _ Black Pen _ Colored Pencil _ Marker _ Gel Pen _ Crayon _ #2 Pencil | Write one word to describe me: |

COLOR THE FACES THAT SHOW HOW I FEEL:

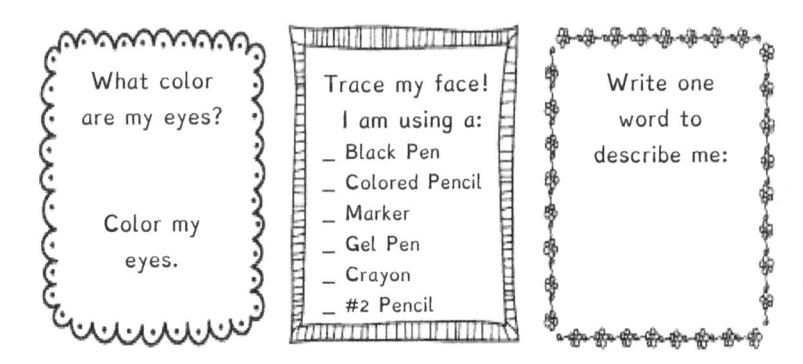

Draw me

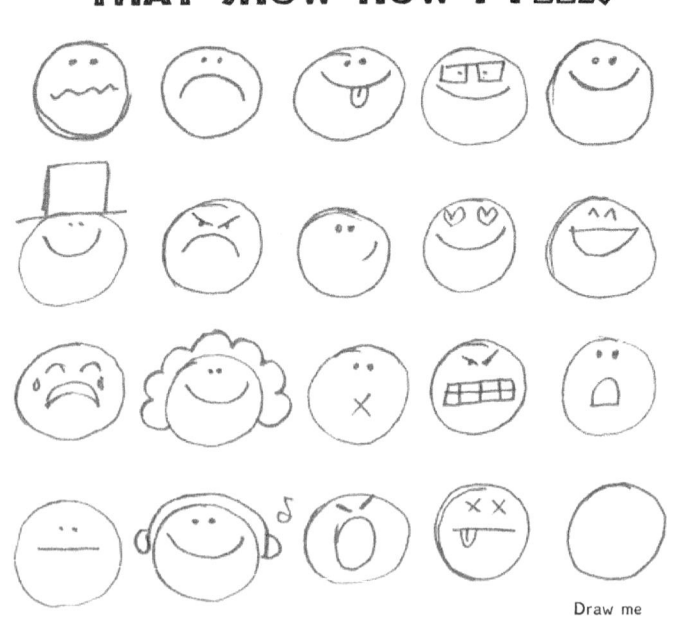

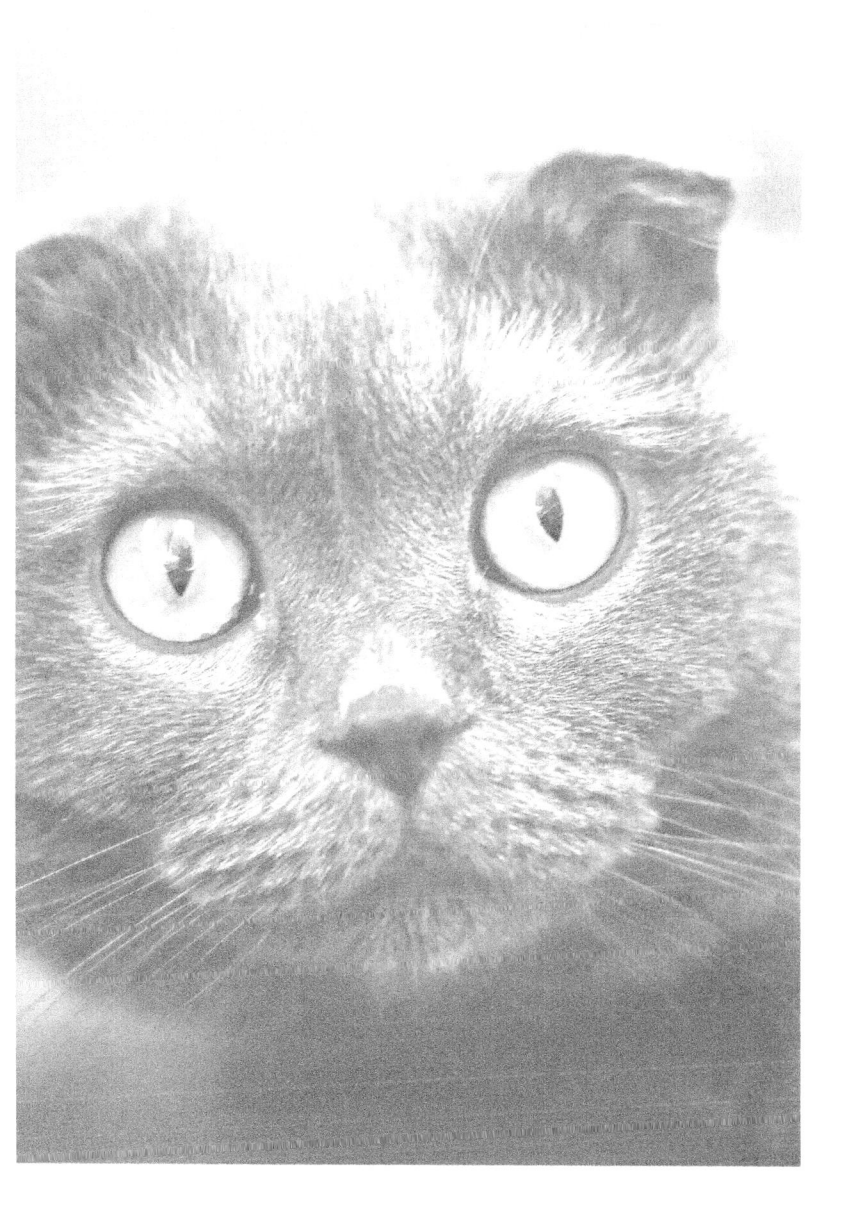

LOOK AT MY FACE!

What color are my eyes?

Color my eyes.

Trace my face!
I am using a:
_ Black Pen
_ Colored Pencil
_ Marker
_ Gel Pen
_ Crayon
_ #2 Pencil

Write one word to describe me:

COLOR THE FACES THAT SHOW HOW I FEEL:

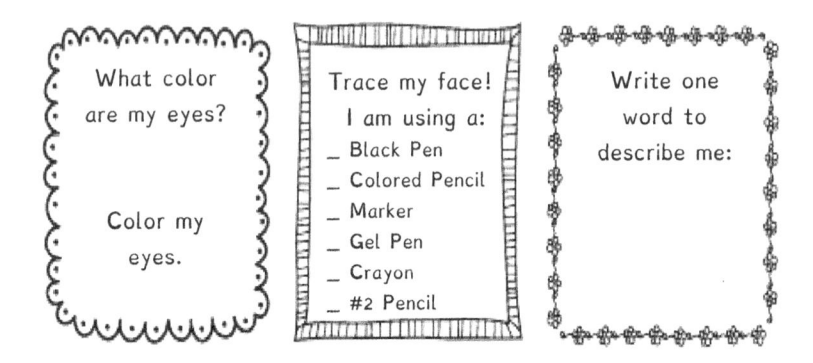

Draw me

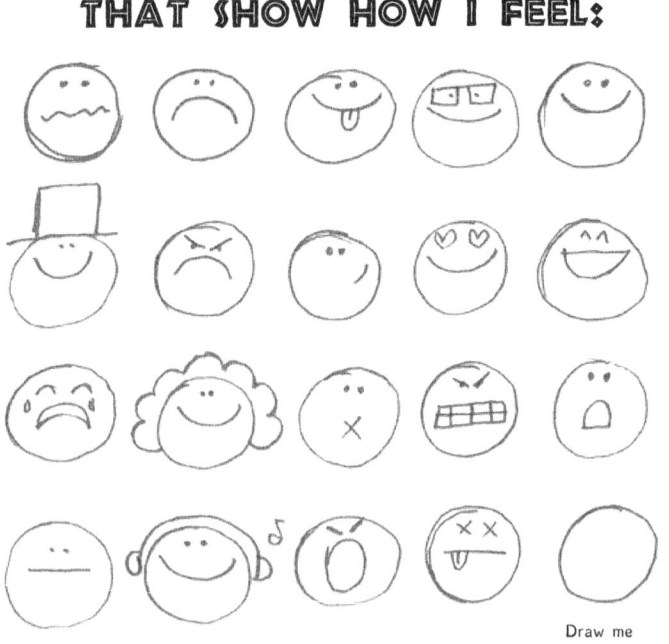

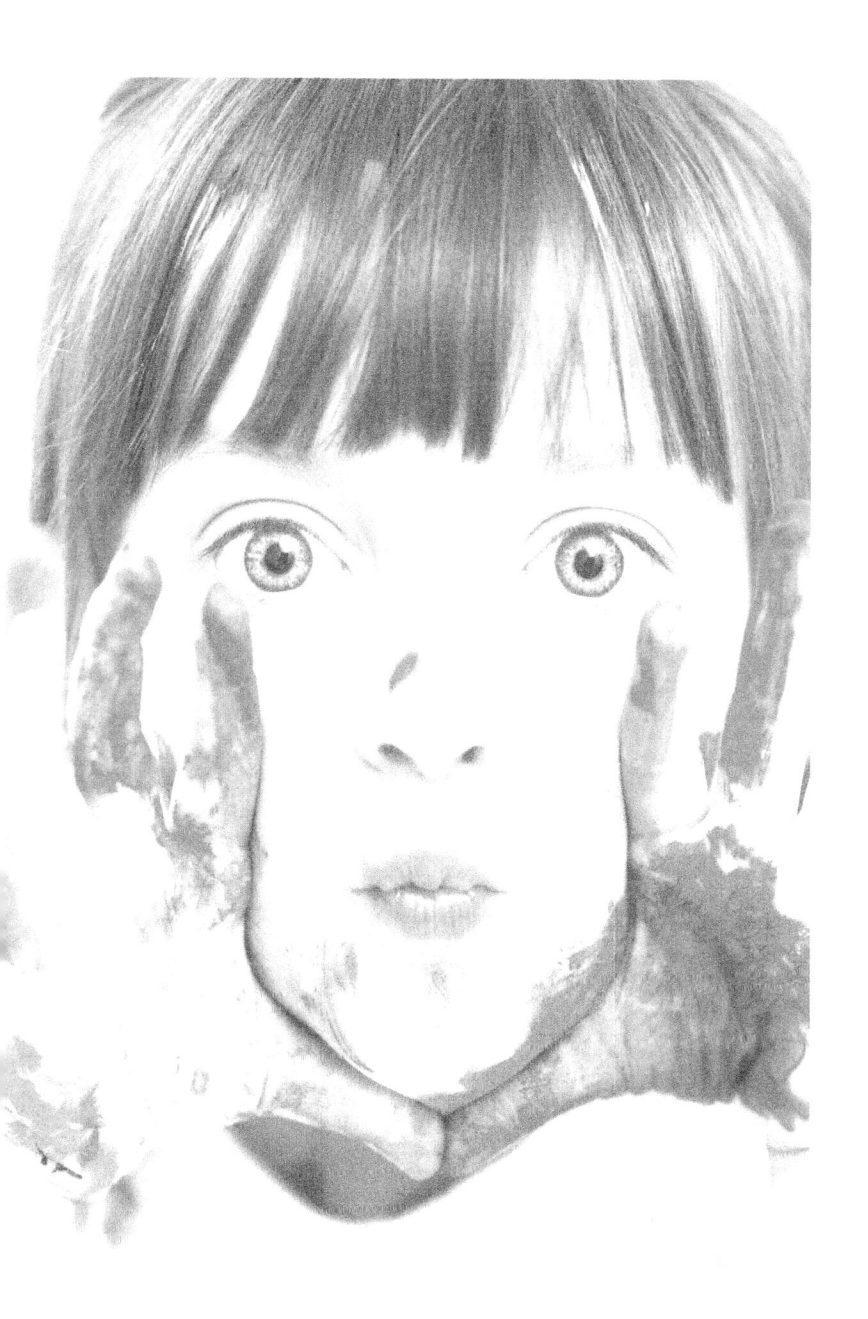

Today I am thinking about:

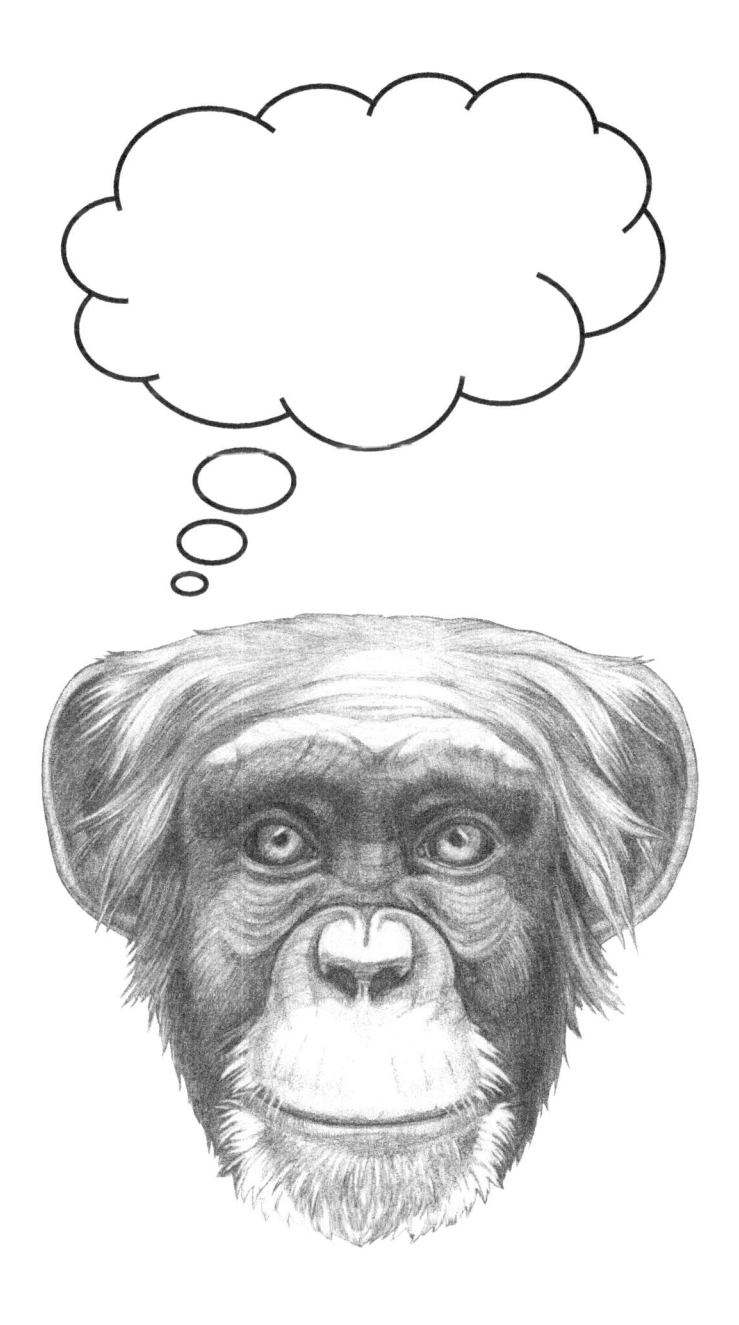

DRAW ANYTHING

LOGIC GAMES

Draw the missing parts of the pattern or design.

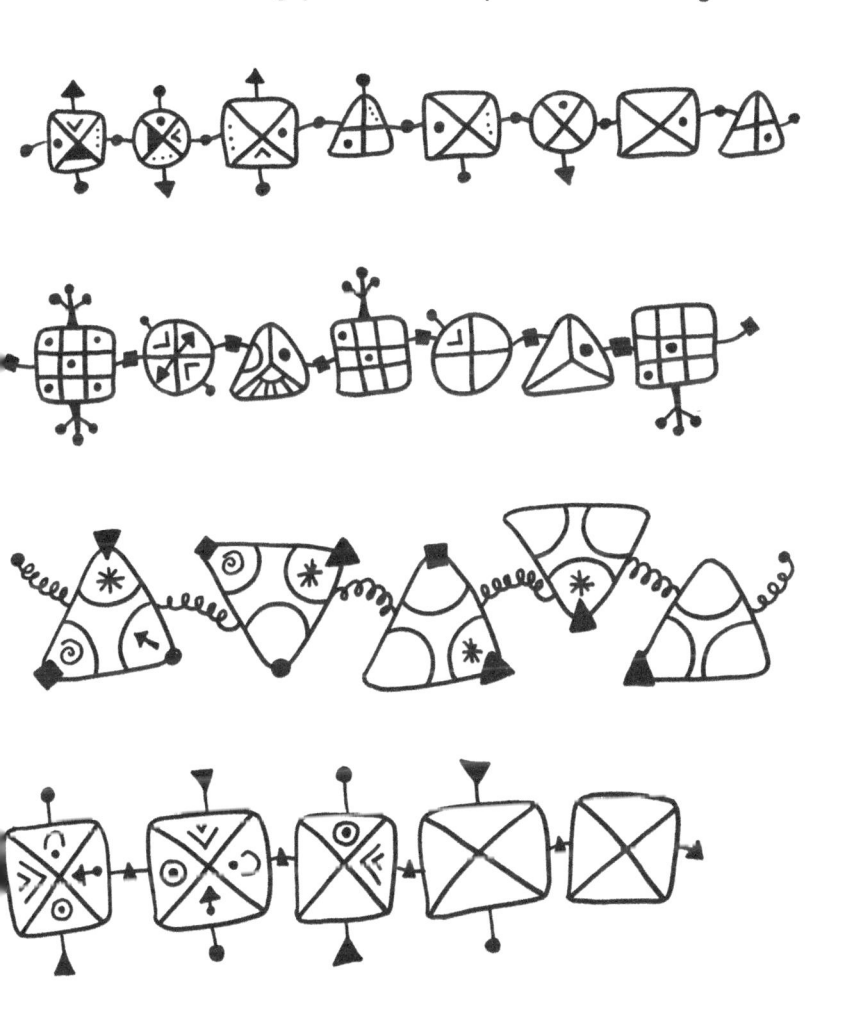

LOOK AT MY FACE!

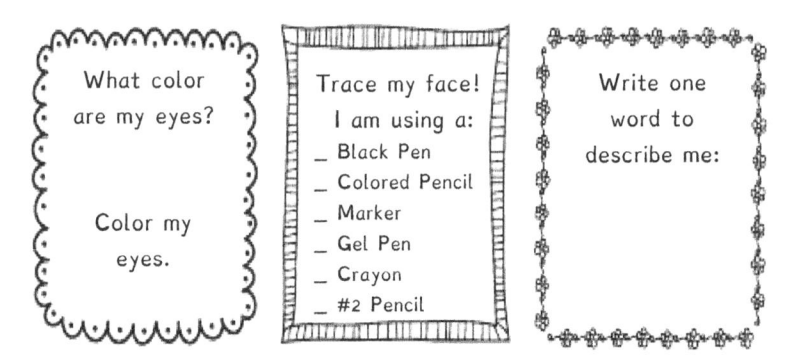

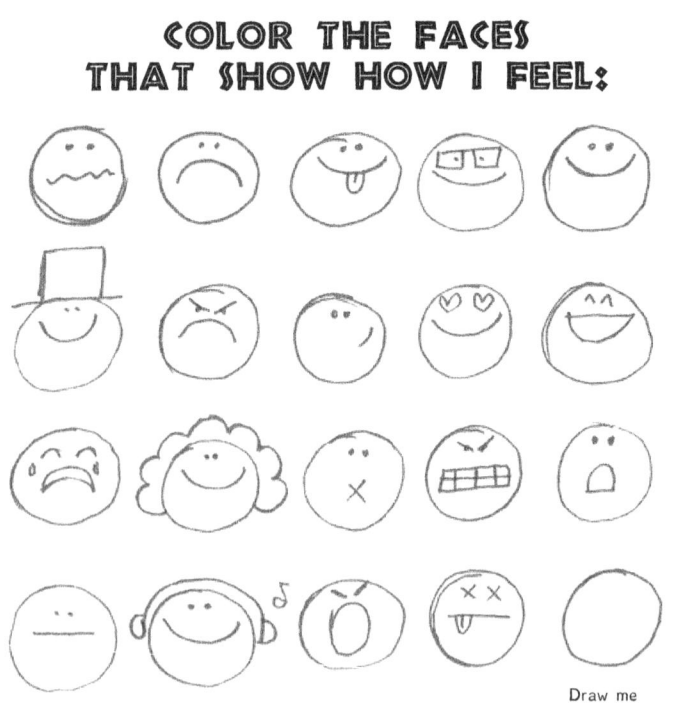

| What color are my eyes? Color my eyes. | Trace my face! I am using a: _ Black Pen _ Colored Pencil _ Marker _ Gel Pen _ Crayon _ #2 Pencil | Write one word to describe me: |

COLOR THE FACES THAT SHOW HOW I FEEL:

Draw me

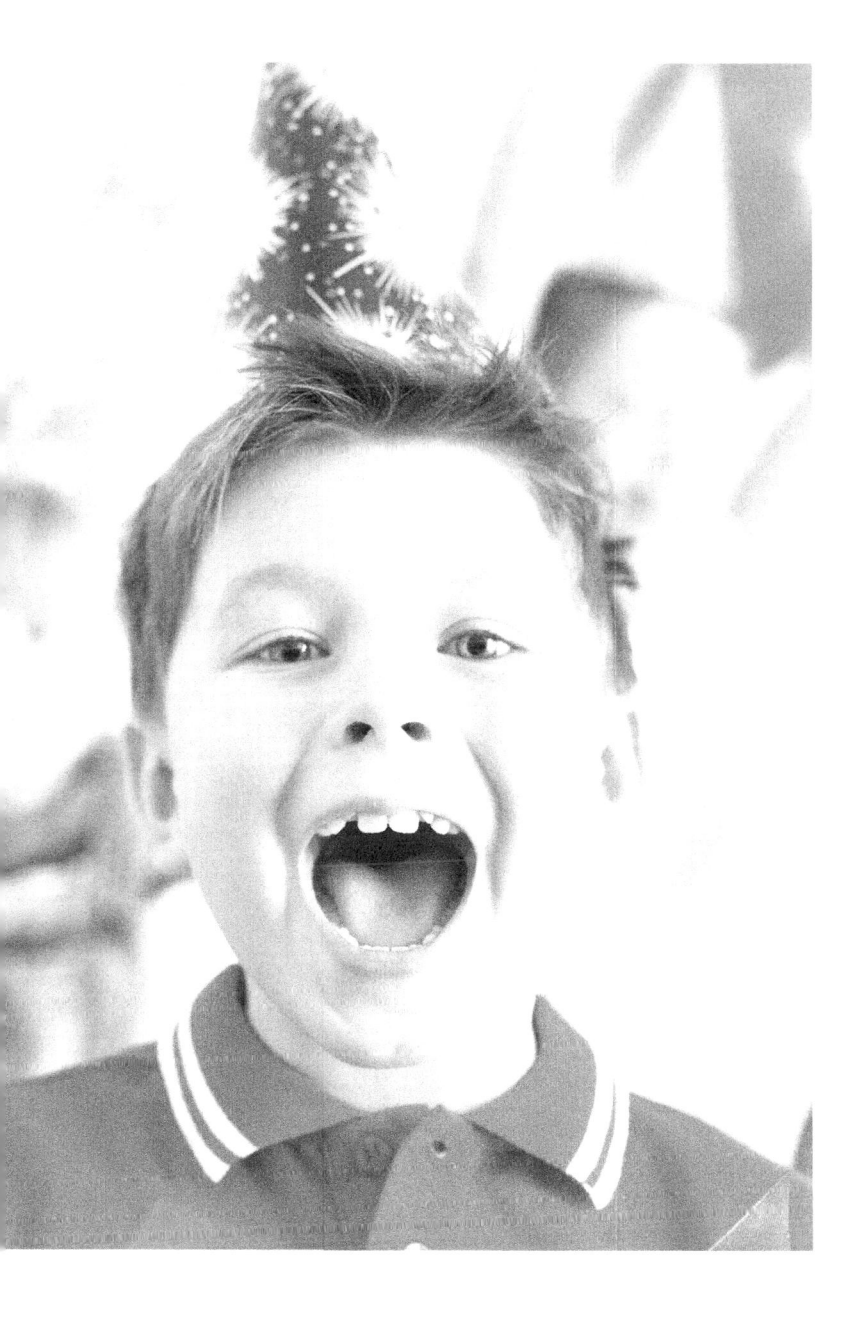

LOOK AT MY FACE!

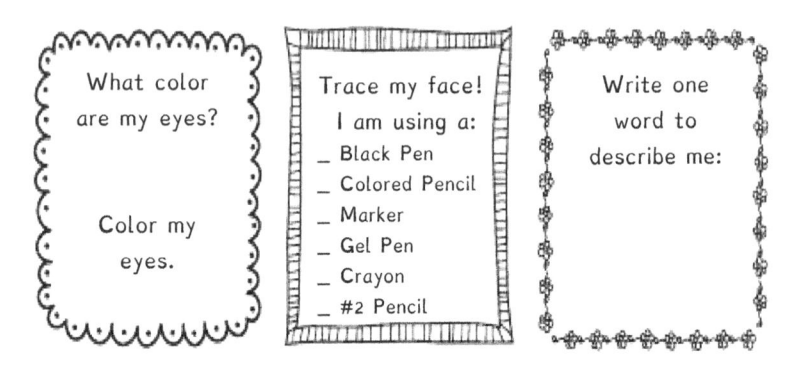

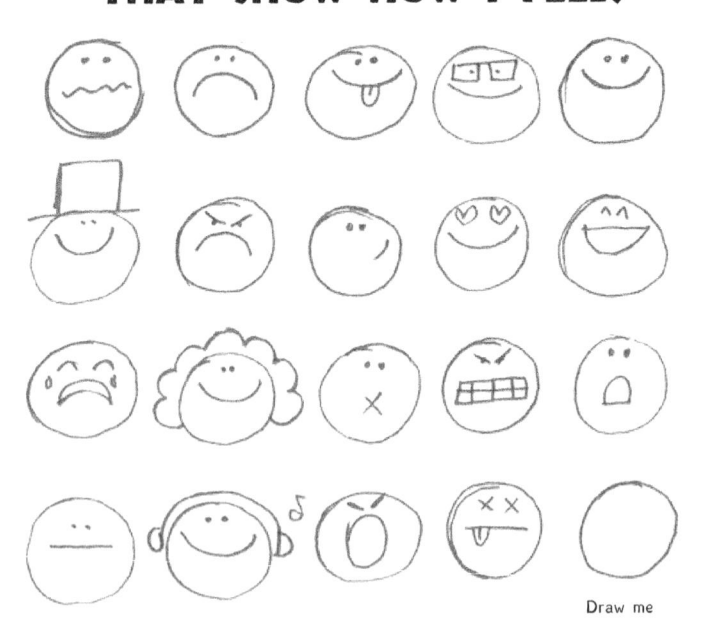

What color are my eyes?

Color my eyes.

Trace my face!
I am using a:
_ Black Pen
_ Colored Pencil
_ Marker
_ Gel Pen
_ Crayon
_ #2 Pencil

Write one word to describe me:

COLOR THE FACES THAT SHOW HOW I FEEL:

Draw me

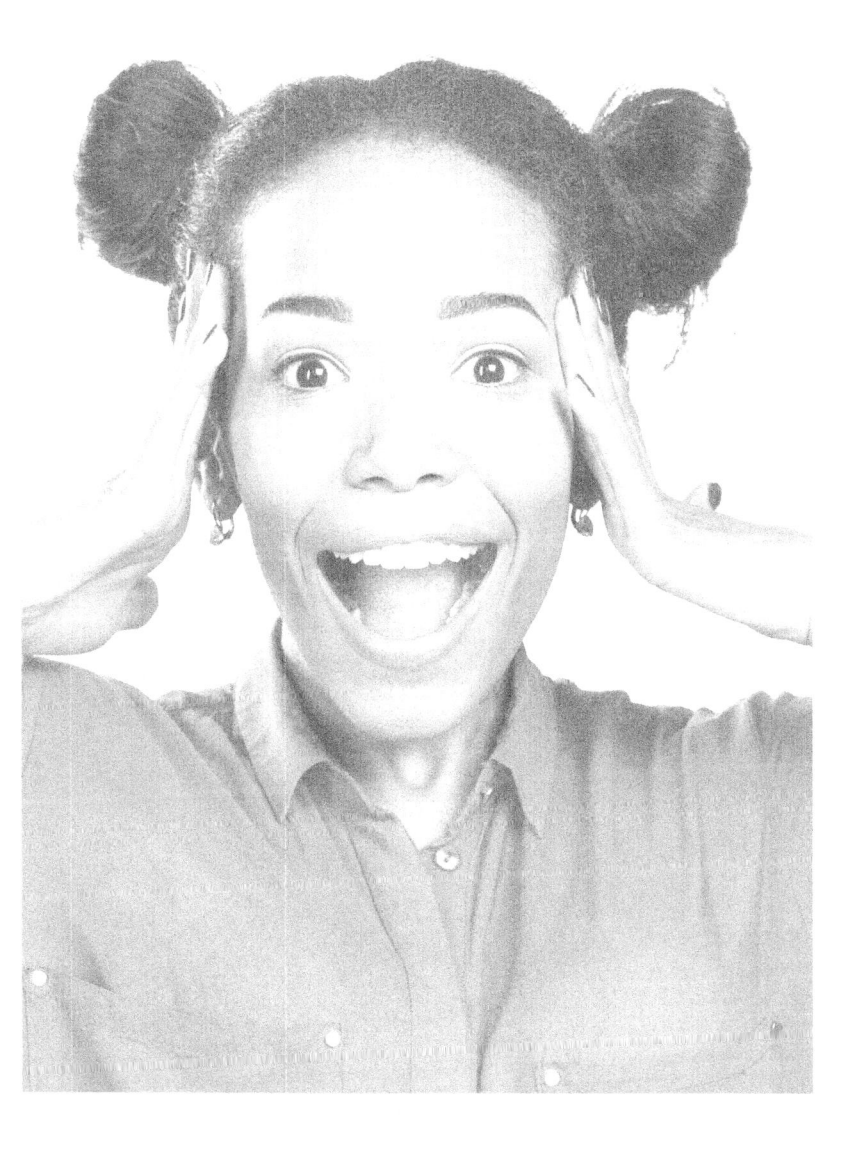

LOOK AT MY FACE!

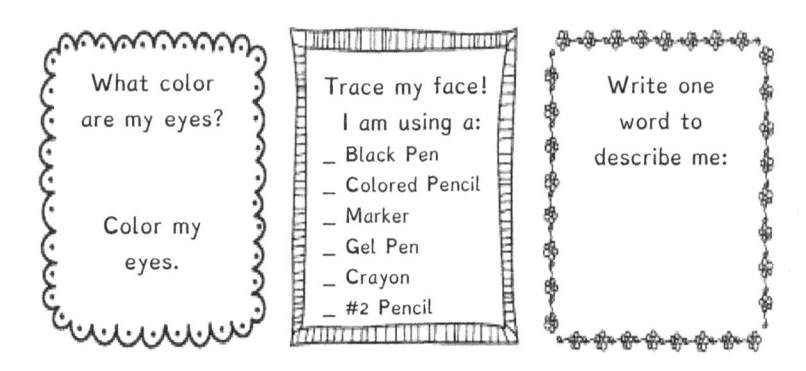

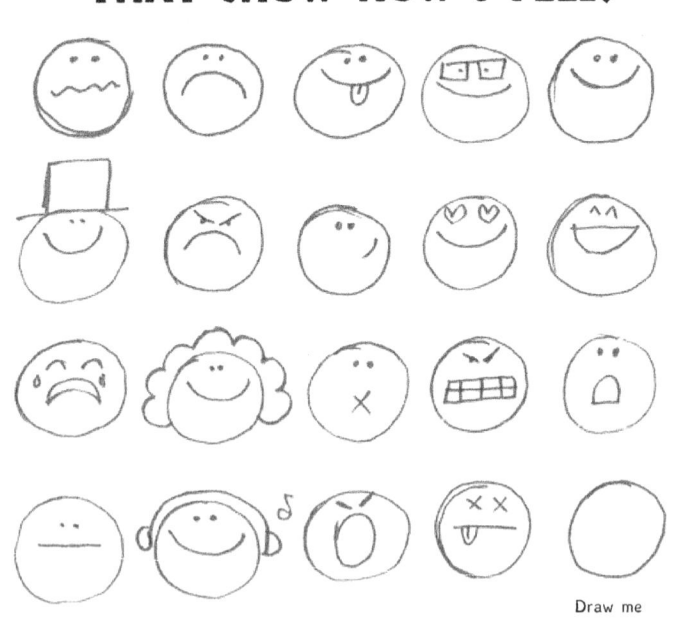

What color are my eyes?

Color my eyes.

Trace my face!
I am using a:
_ Black Pen
_ Colored Pencil
_ Marker
_ Gel Pen
_ Crayon
_ #2 Pencil

Write one word to describe me:

COLOR THE FACES THAT SHOW HOW I FEEL:

Draw me

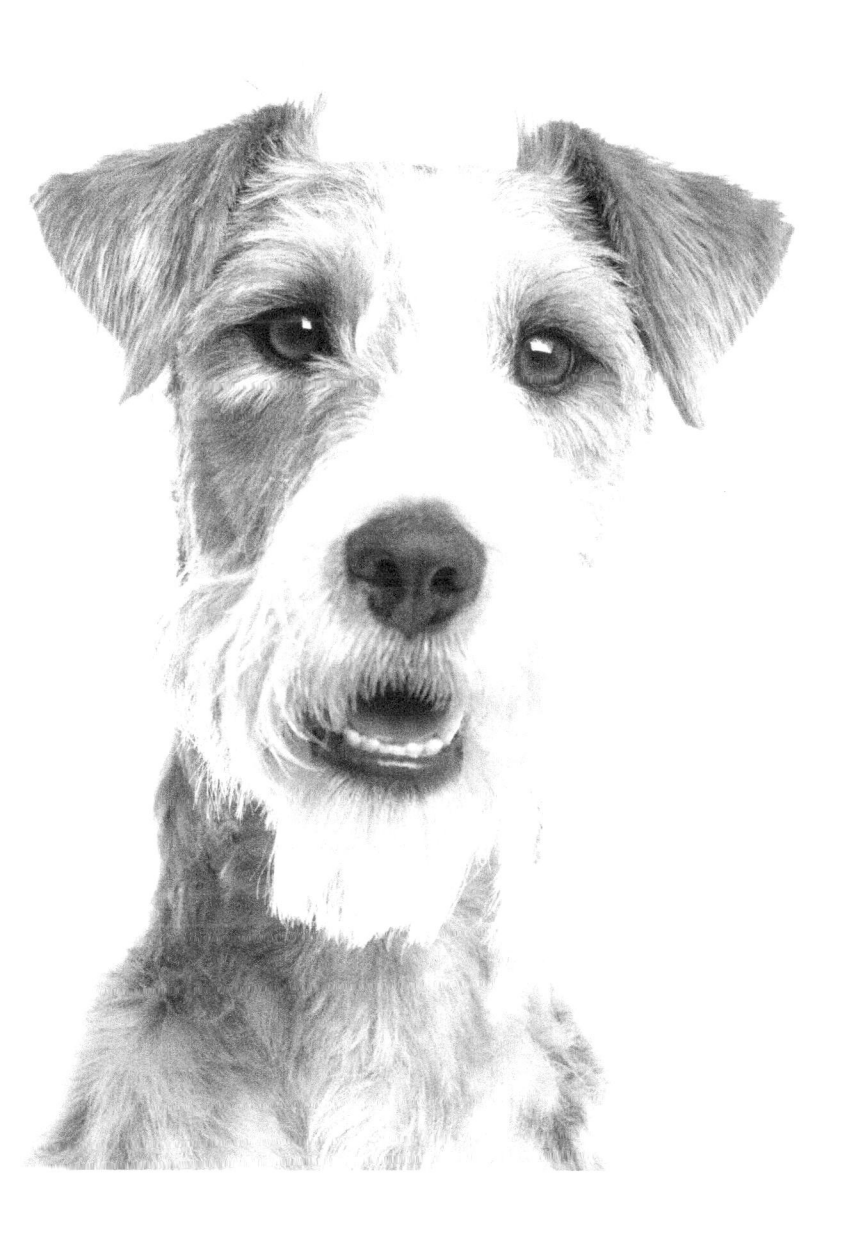

LOOK AT MY FACE!

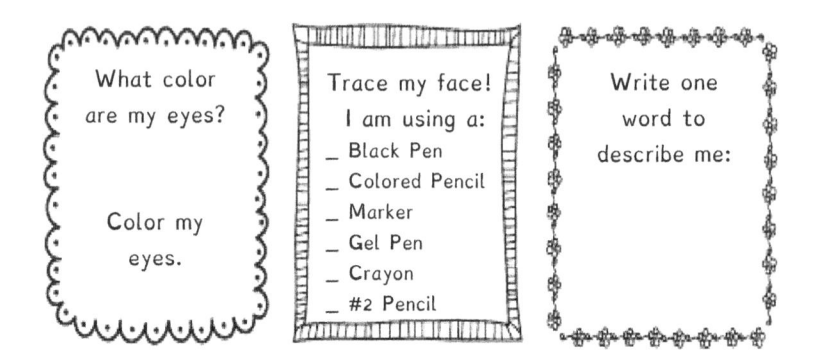

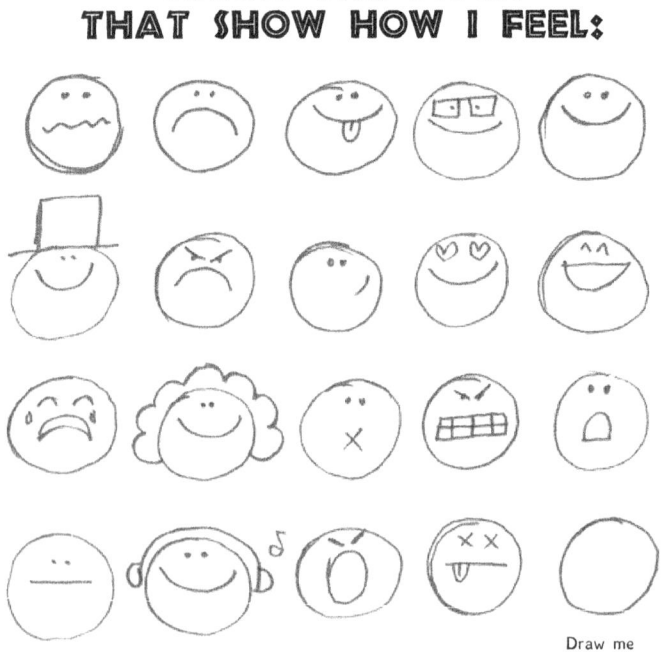

> What color are my eyes?
>
> Color my eyes.

> Trace my face!
> I am using a:
> _ Black Pen
> _ Colored Pencil
> _ Marker
> _ Gel Pen
> _ Crayon
> _ #2 Pencil

> Write one word to describe me:

COLOR THE FACES THAT SHOW HOW I FEEL:

Draw me

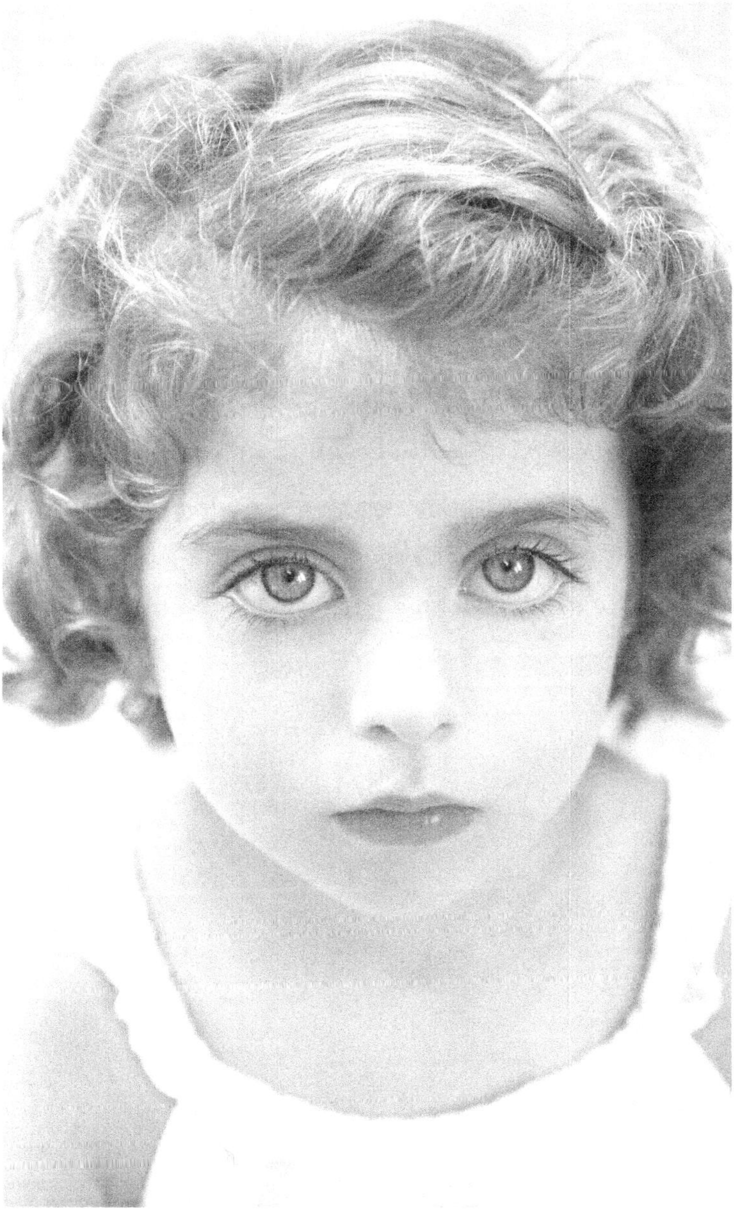

LOOK AT MY FACE!

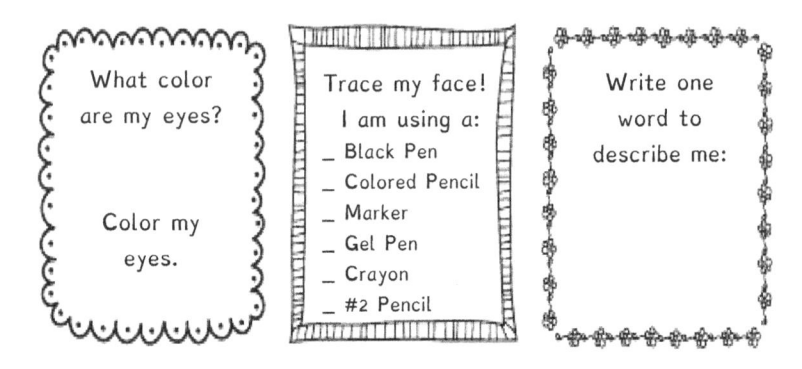

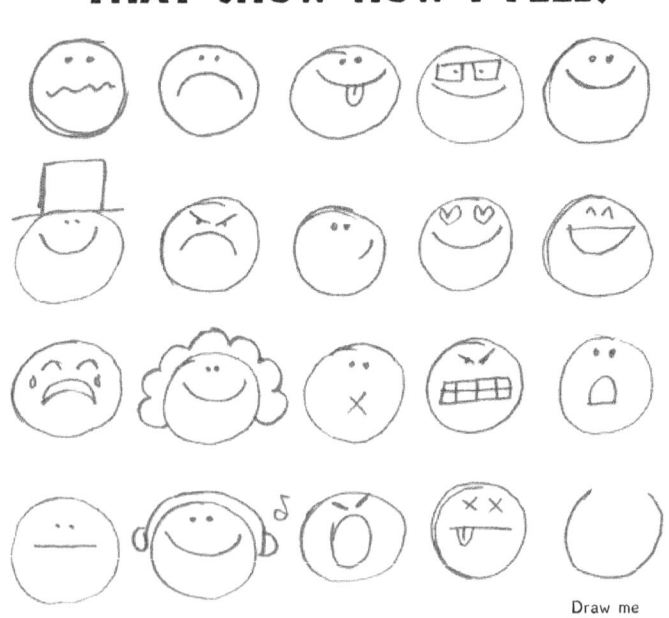

What color are my eyes? Color my eyes.	Trace my face! I am using a: _ Black Pen _ Colored Pencil _ Marker _ Gel Pen _ Crayon _ #2 Pencil	Write one word to describe me:

COLOR THE FACES THAT SHOW HOW I FEEL:

Draw me

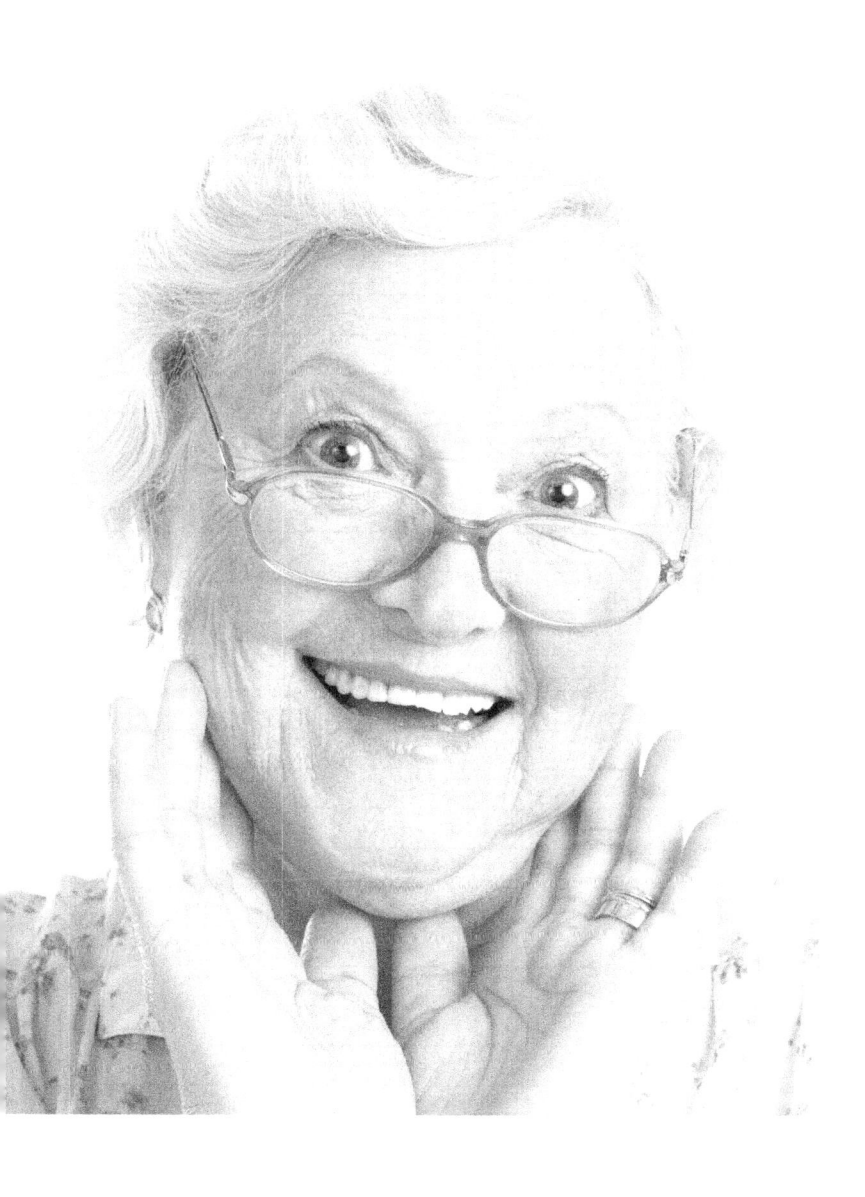

Today I am thinking about:

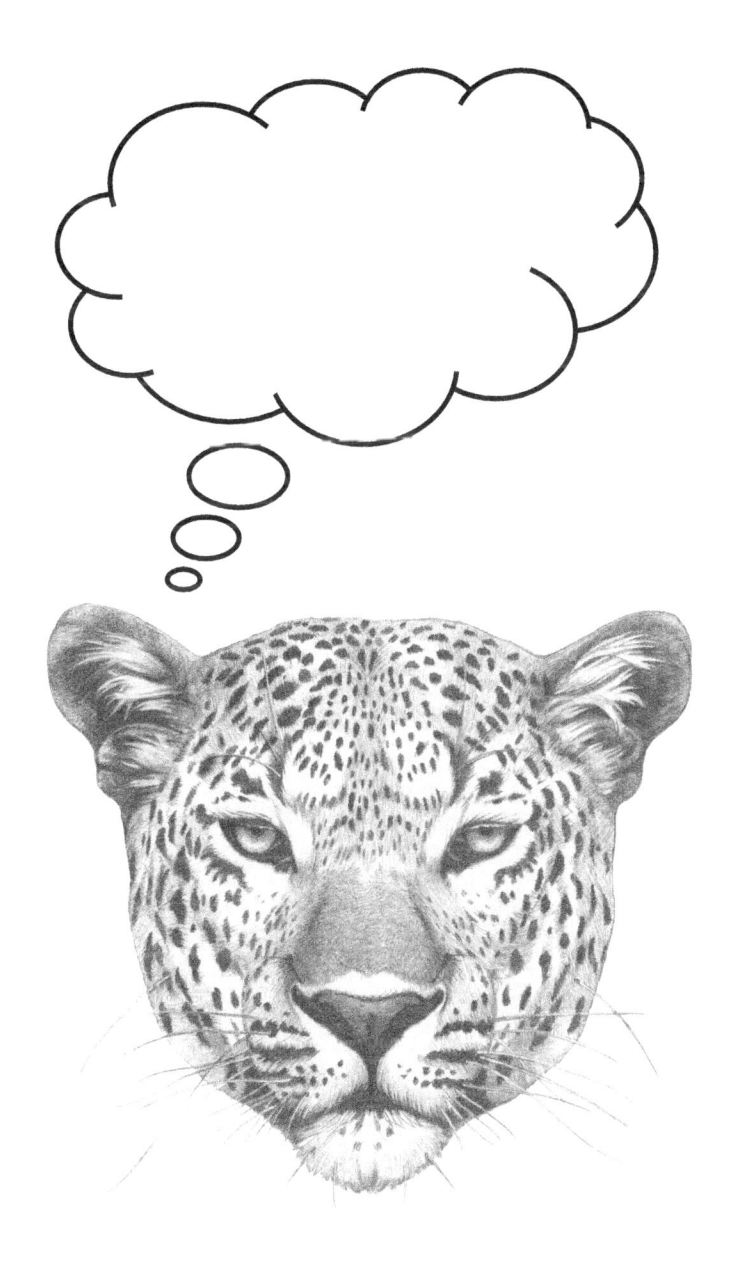

DRAW ANYTHING

LOGIC GAMES

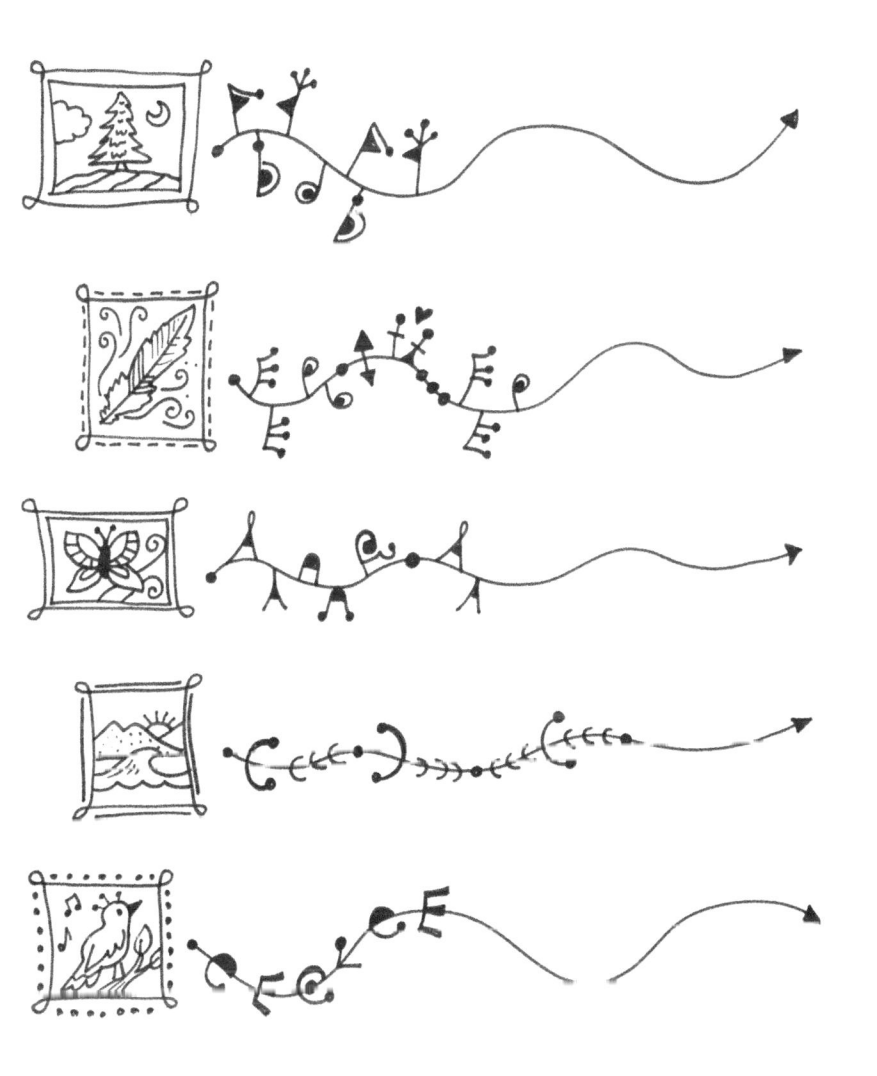

LOOK AT MY FACE!

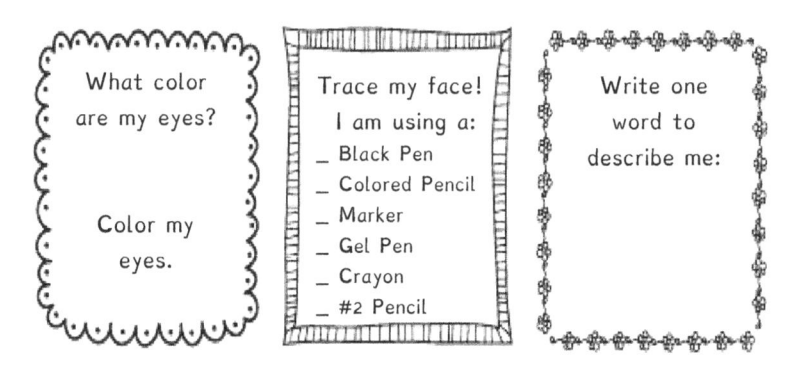

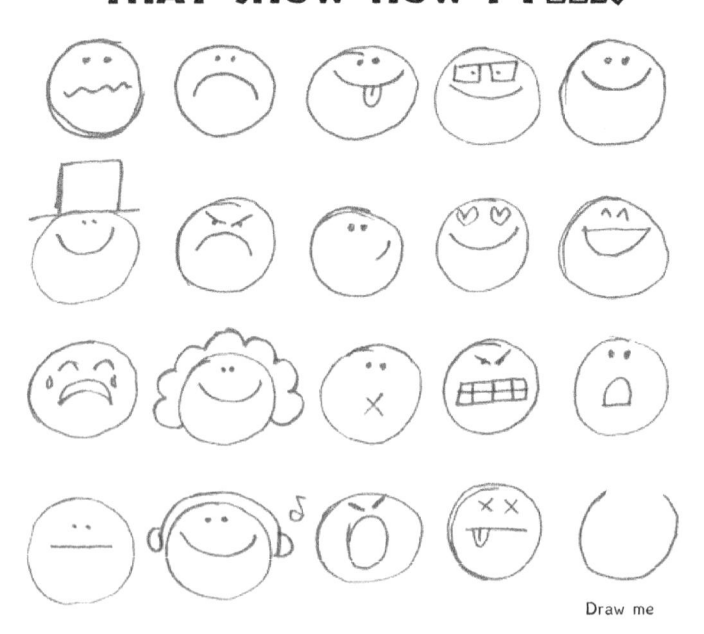

What color are my eyes?

Color my eyes.

Trace my face!
I am using a:
_ Black Pen
_ Colored Pencil
_ Marker
_ Gel Pen
_ Crayon
_ #2 Pencil

Write one word to describe me:

COLOR THE FACES THAT SHOW HOW I FEEL:

Draw me

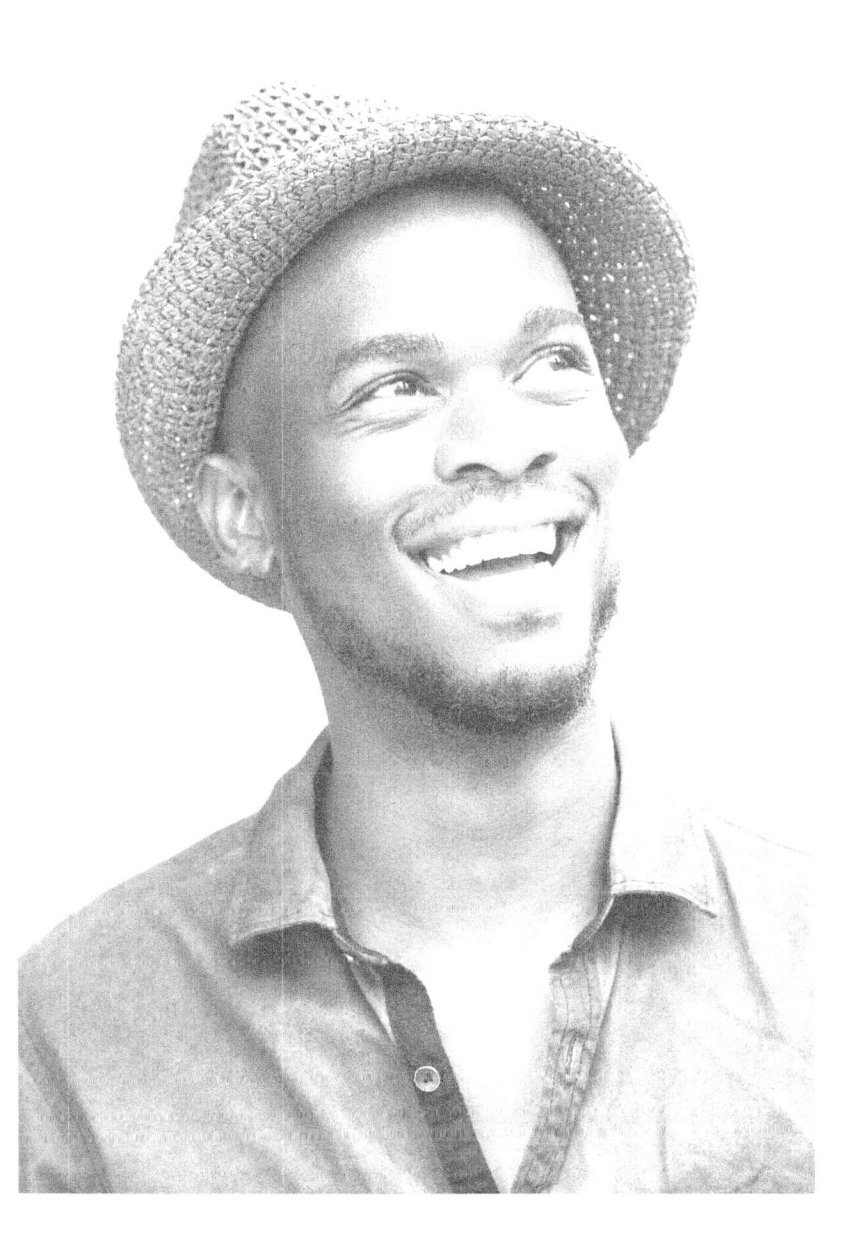

LOOK AT MY FACE!

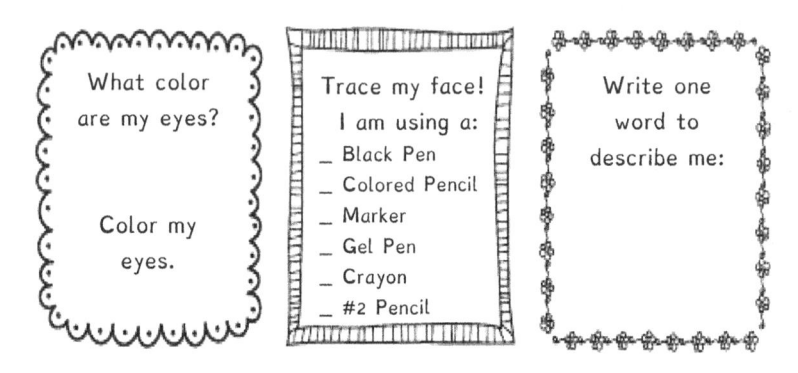

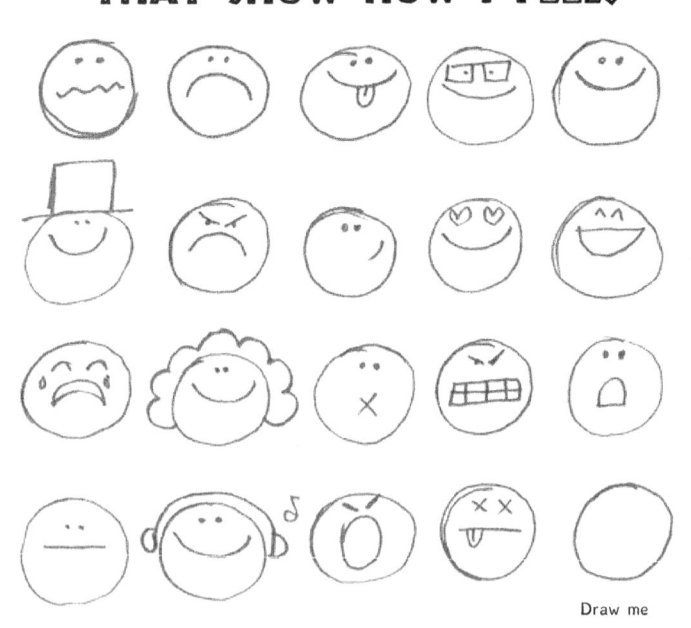

What color are my eyes?

Color my eyes.

Trace my face!
I am using a:
_ Black Pen
_ Colored Pencil
_ Marker
_ Gel Pen
_ Crayon
_ #2 Pencil

Write one word to describe me:

COLOR THE FACES THAT SHOW HOW I FEEL:

Draw me

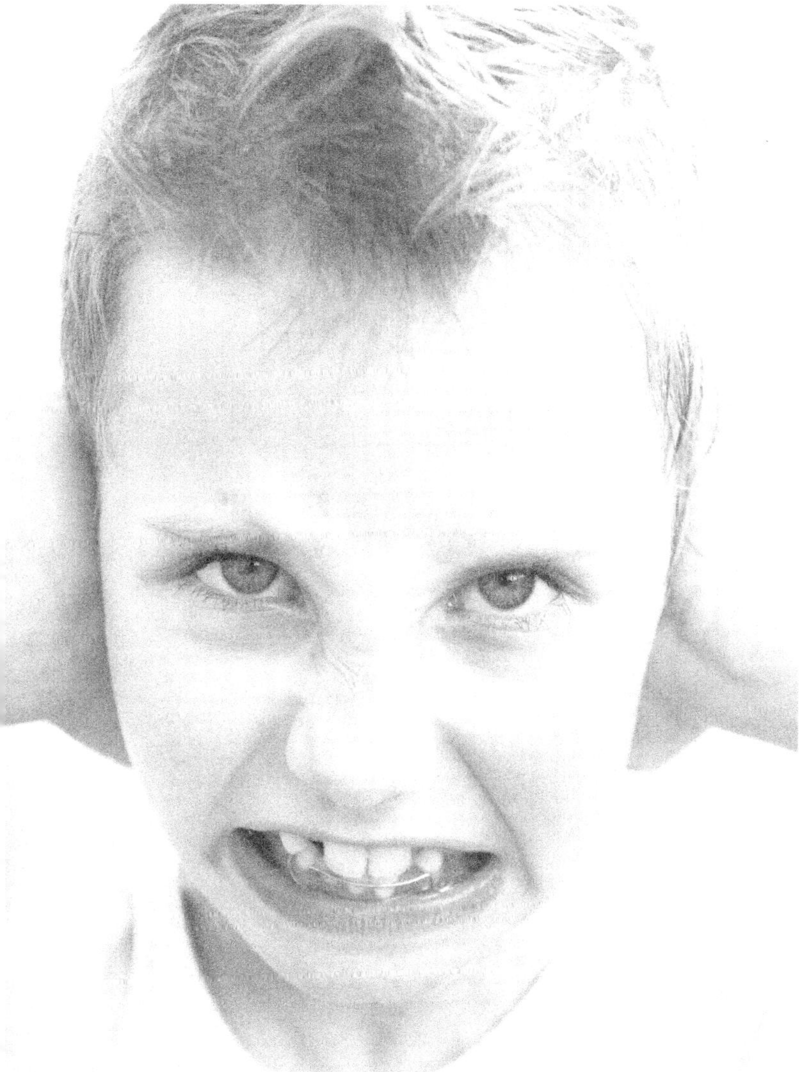

LOOK AT MY FACE!

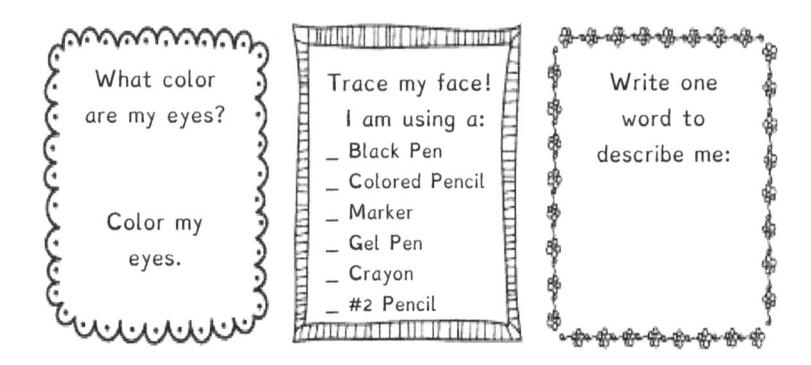

What color are my eyes?

Color my eyes.

Trace my face!
I am using a:
_ Black Pen
_ Colored Pencil
_ Marker
_ Gel Pen
_ Crayon
_ #2 Pencil

Write one word to describe me:

COLOR THE FACES THAT SHOW HOW I FEEL:

Draw me

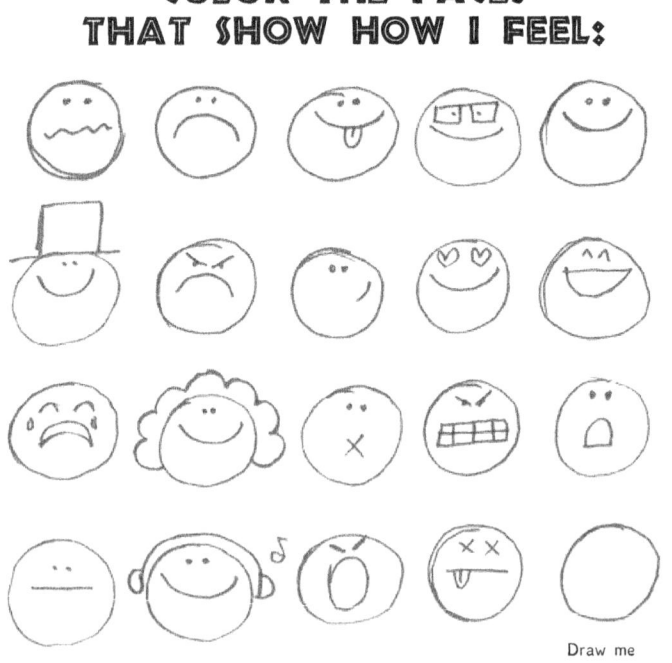

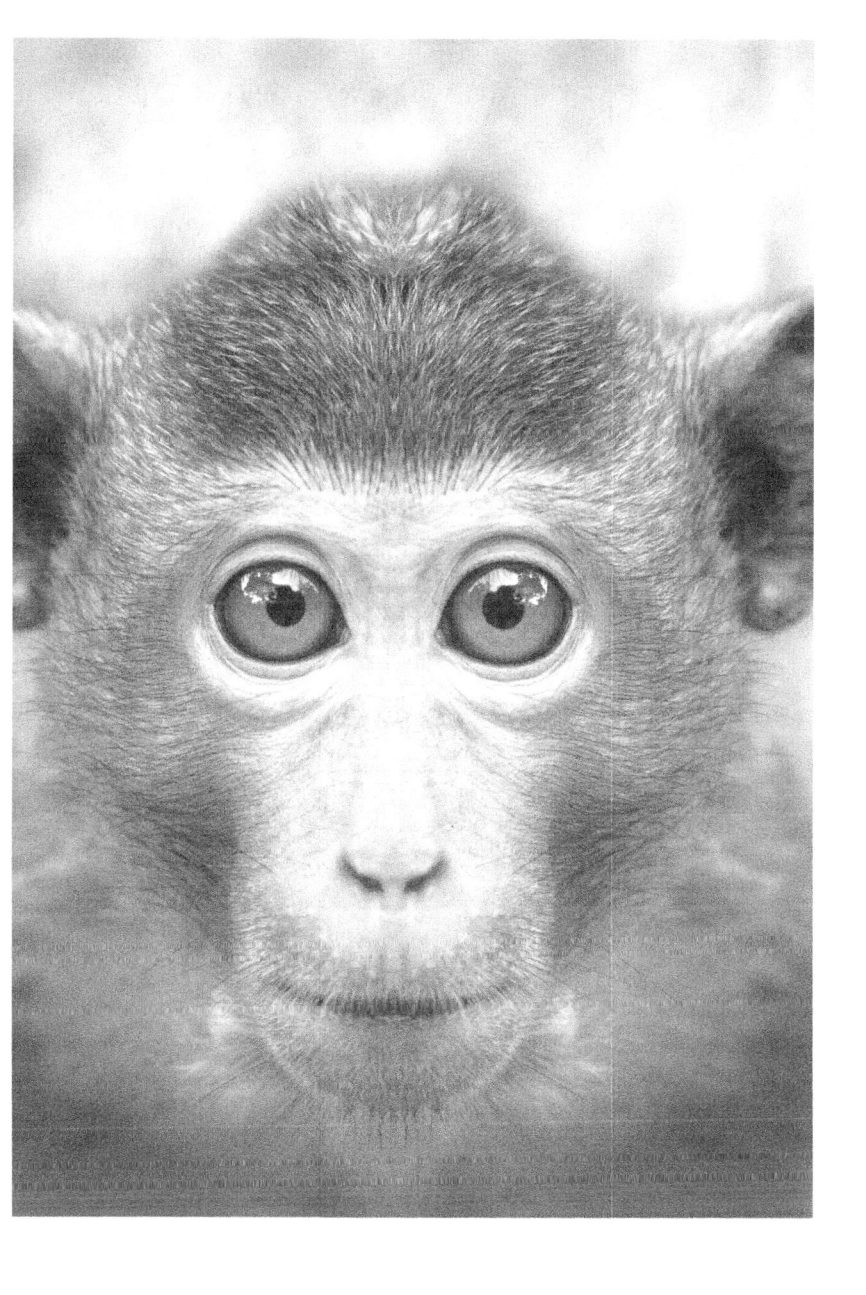

LOOK AT MY FACE!

What color are my eyes?

Color my eyes.

Trace my face!
I am using a:
_ Black Pen
_ Colored Pencil
_ Marker
_ Gel Pen
_ Crayon
_ #2 Pencil

Write one word to describe me:

COLOR THE FACES THAT SHOW HOW I FEEL:

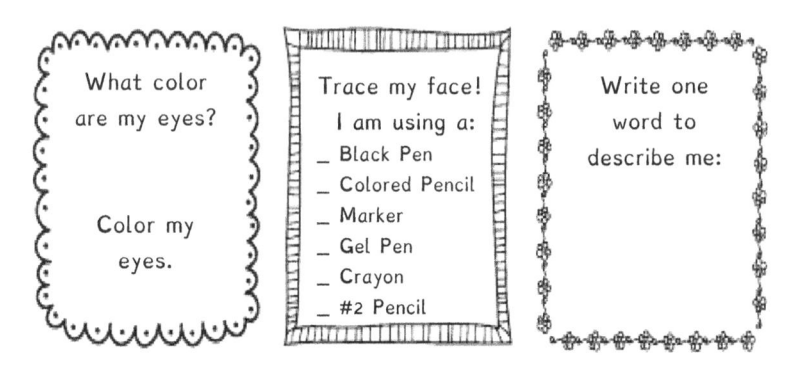

Draw me

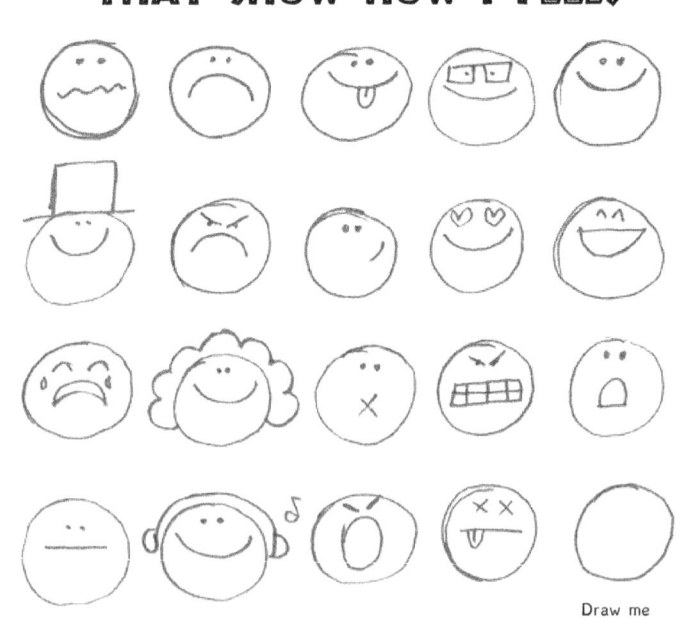

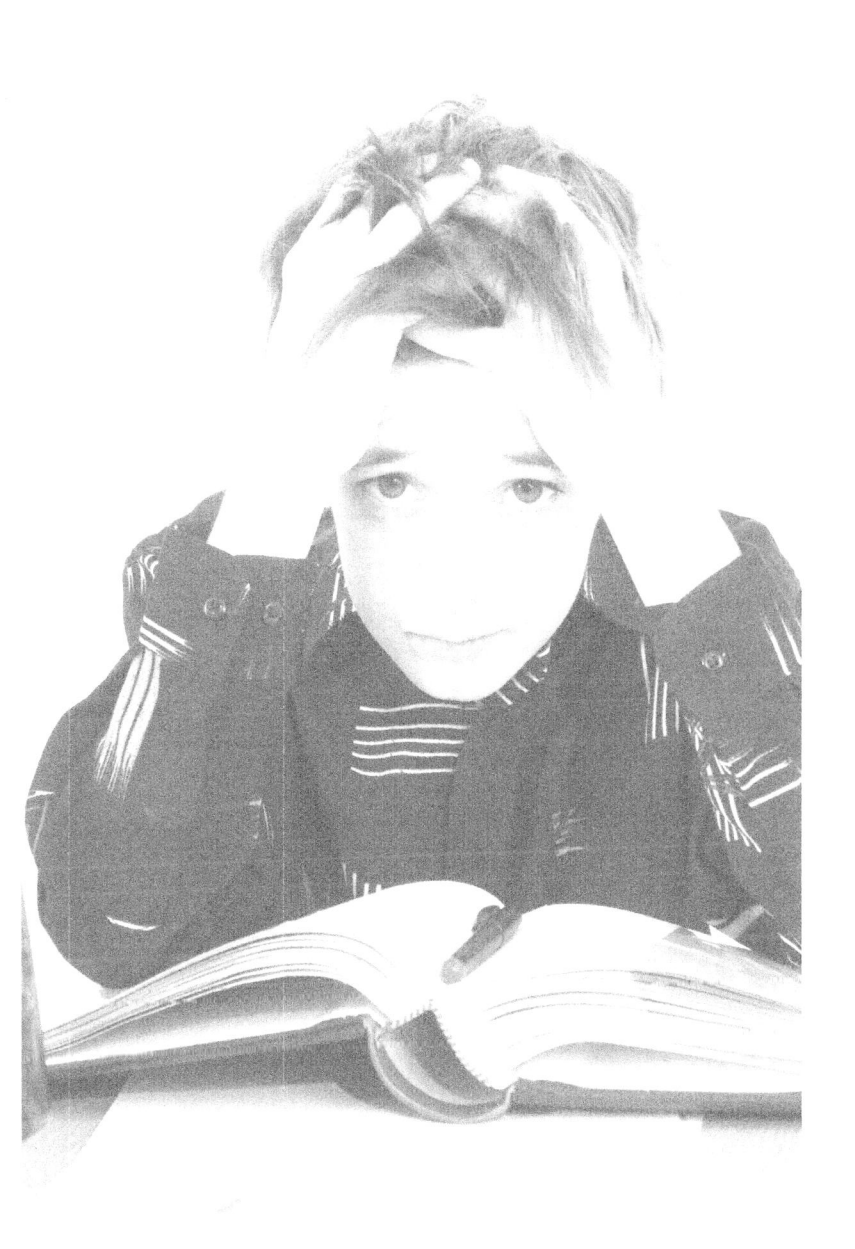

LOOK AT MY FACE!

What color are my eyes?

Color my eyes.

Trace my face!
I am using a:
- _ Black Pen
- _ Colored Pencil
- _ Marker
- _ Gel Pen
- _ Crayon
- _ #2 Pencil

Write one word to describe me:

COLOR THE FACES THAT SHOW HOW I FEEL:

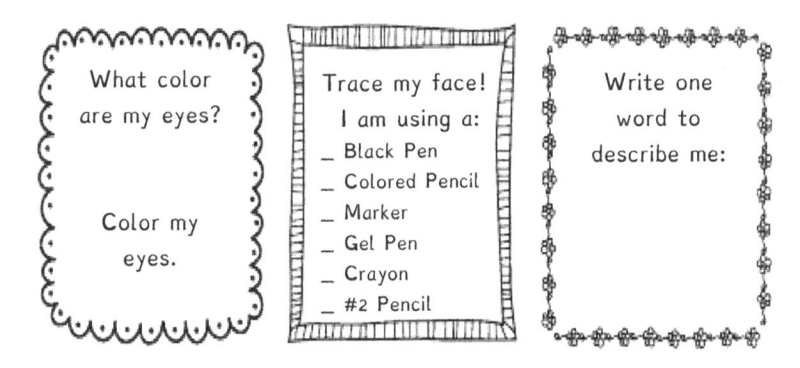

Draw me

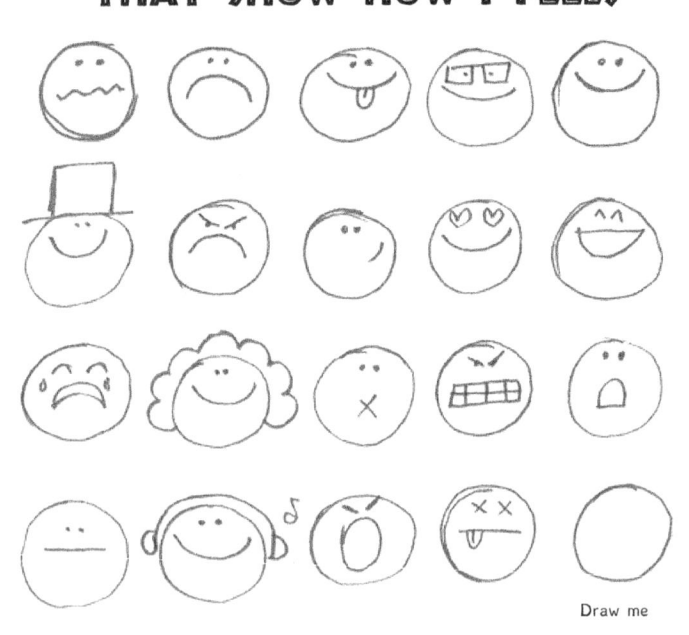

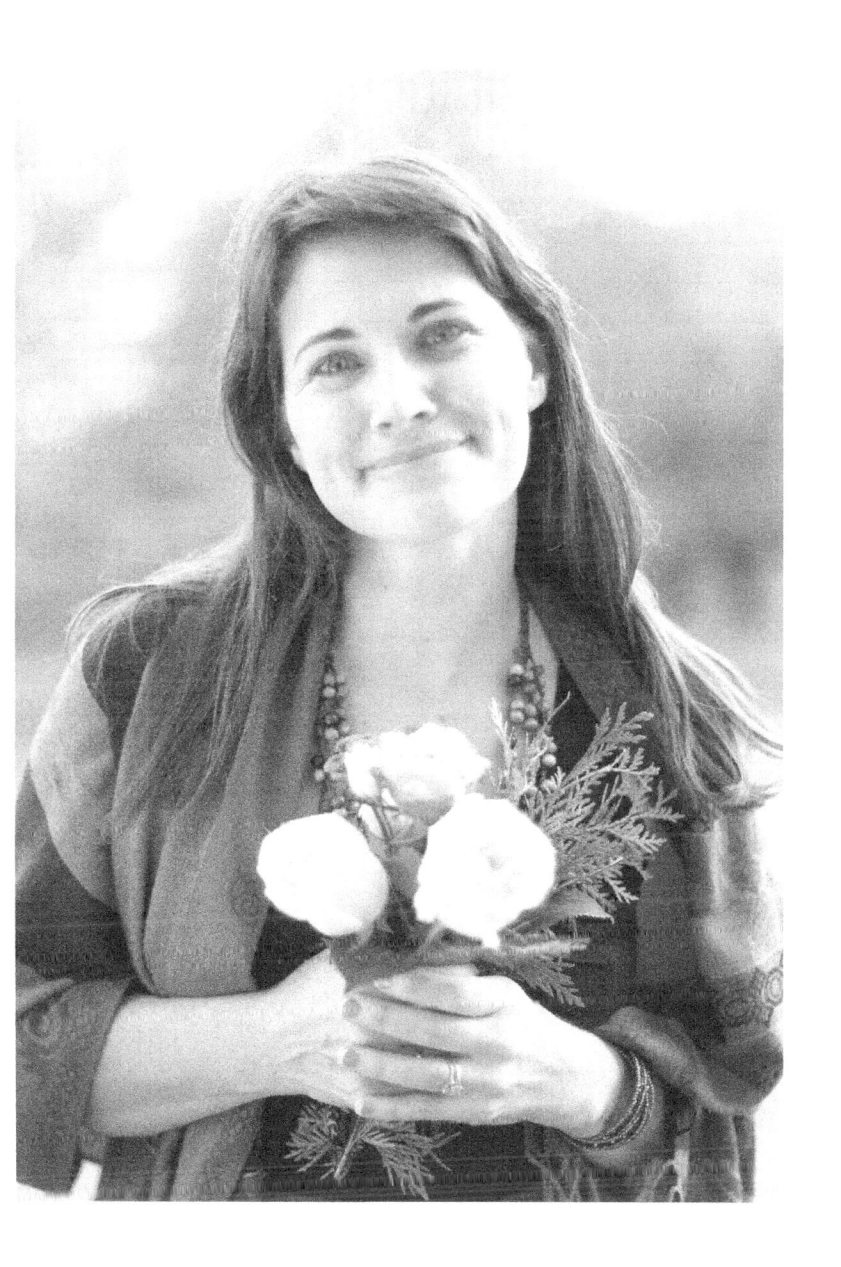

Today I am thinking about:

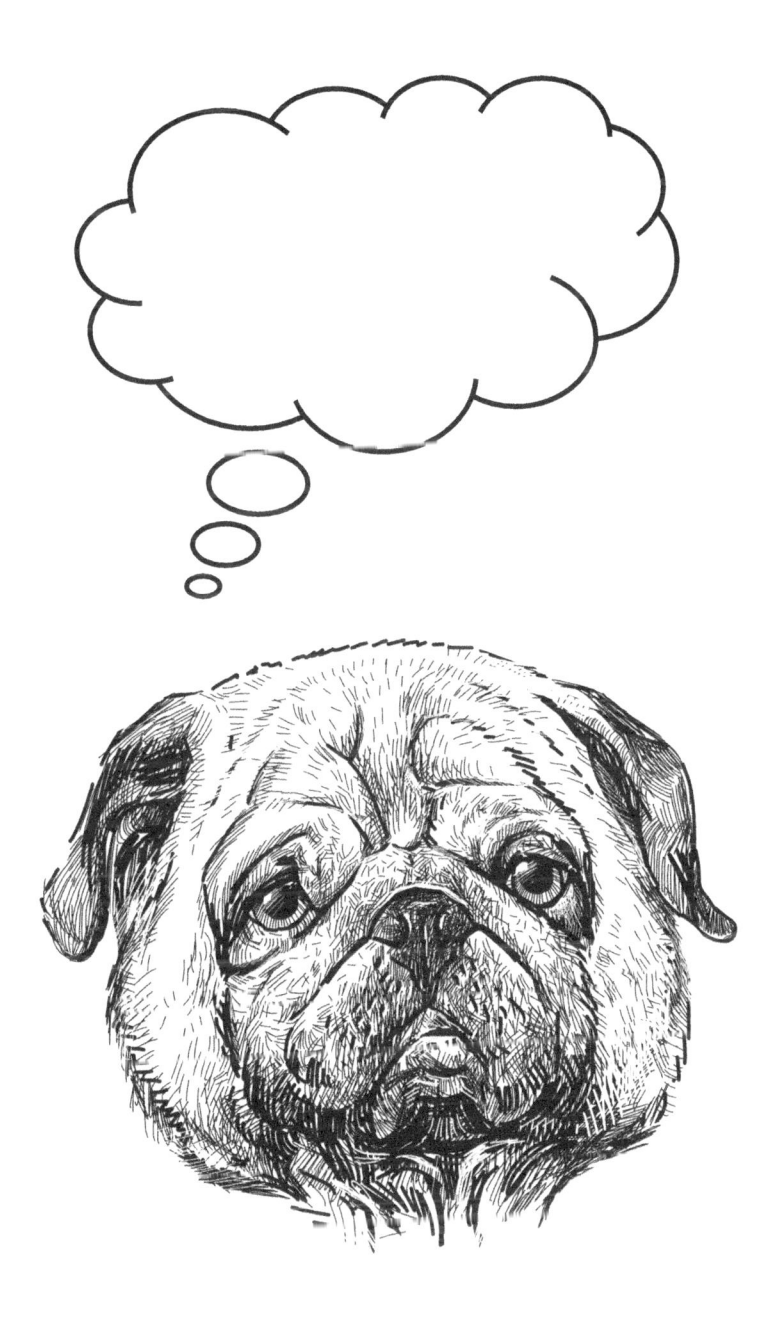

DRAW ANYTHING

LOGIC GAMES

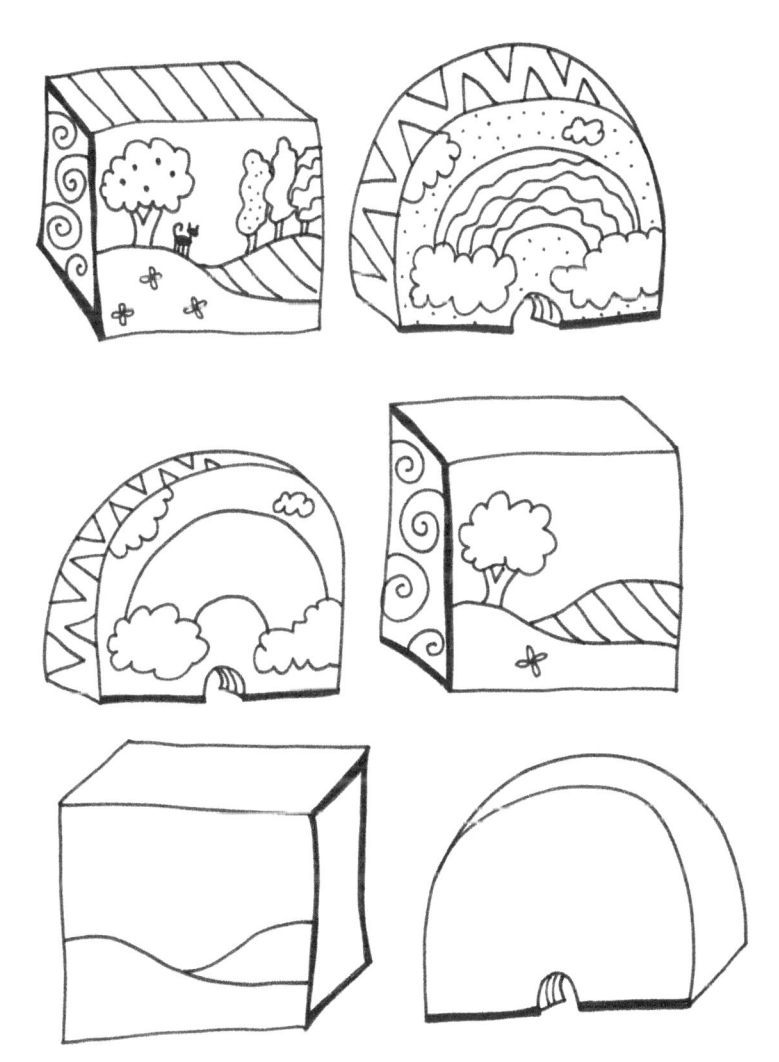

LOOK AT MY FACE!

What color are my eyes?

Color my eyes.

Trace my face!
I am using a:
- Black Pen
- Colored Pencil
- Marker
- Gel Pen
- Crayon
- #2 Pencil

Write one word to describe me:

COLOR THE FACES THAT SHOW HOW I FEEL:

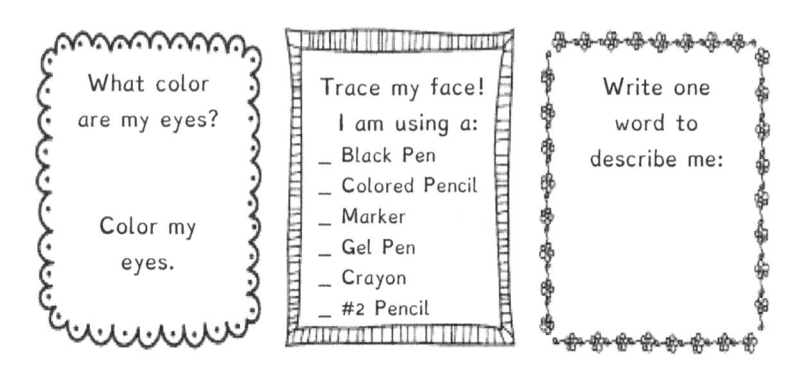

Draw me

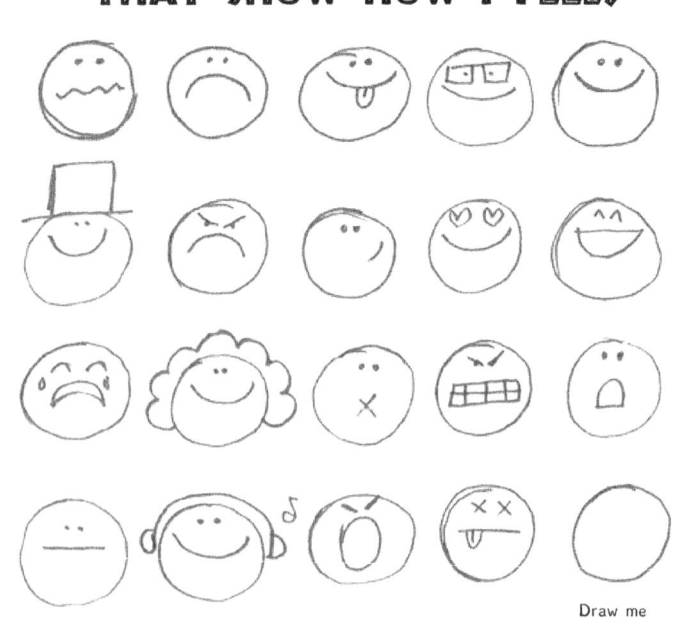

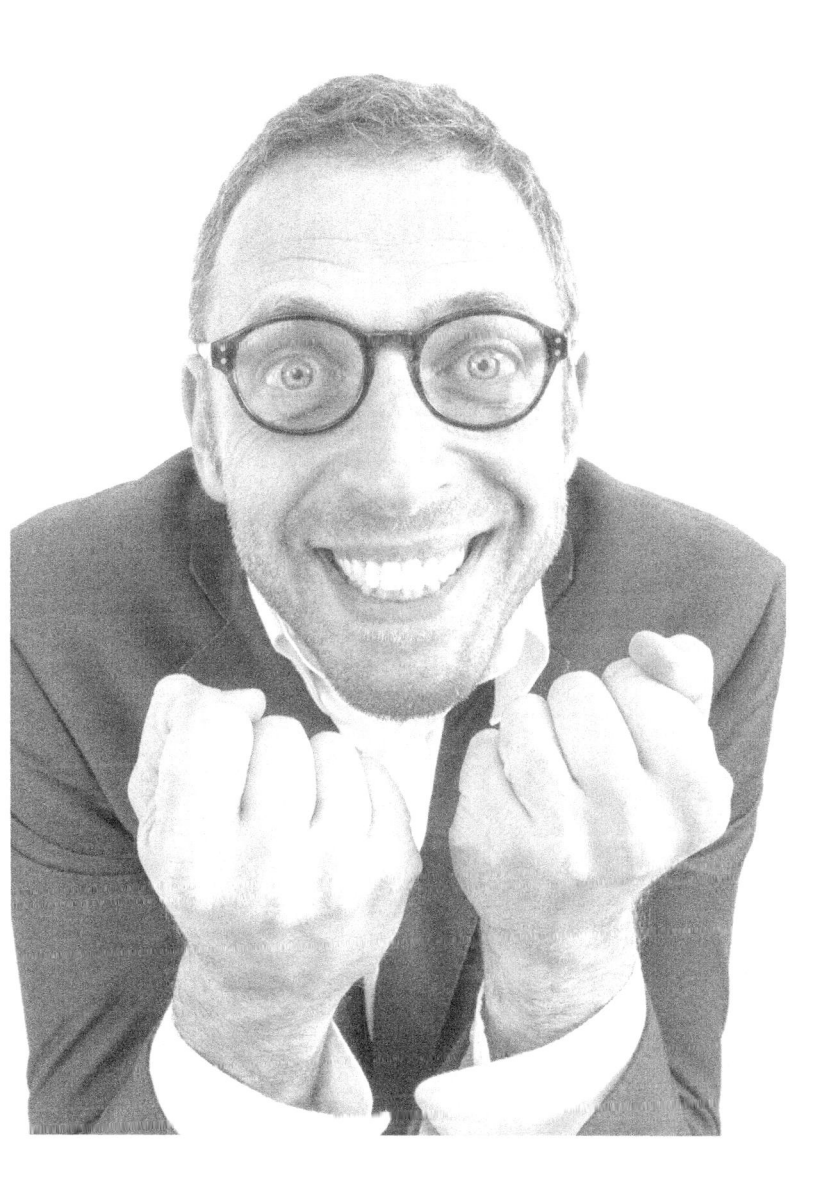

LOOK AT MY FACE!

What color are my eyes?

Color my eyes.

Trace my face!
I am using a:
_ Black Pen
_ Colored Pencil
_ Marker
_ Gel Pen
_ Crayon
_ #2 Pencil

Write one word to describe me:

COLOR THE FACES THAT SHOW HOW I FEEL:

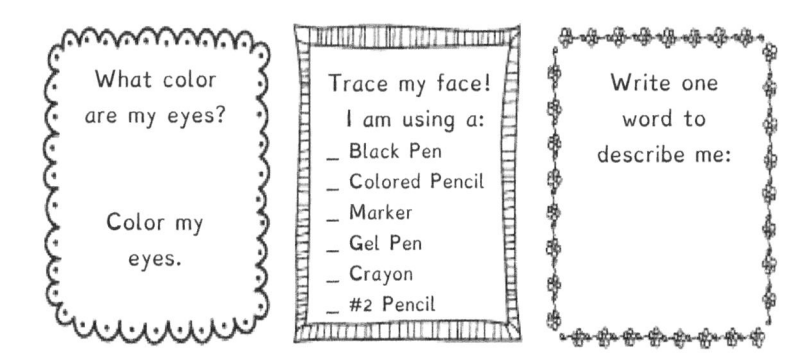

Draw me

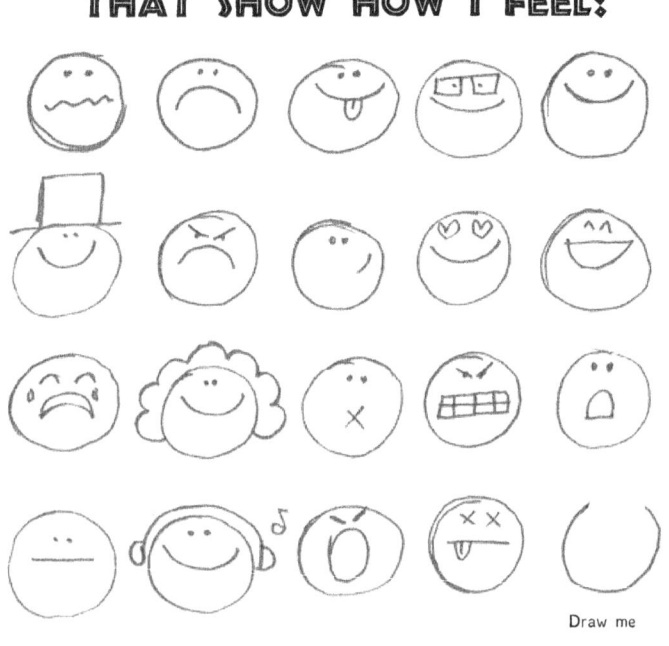

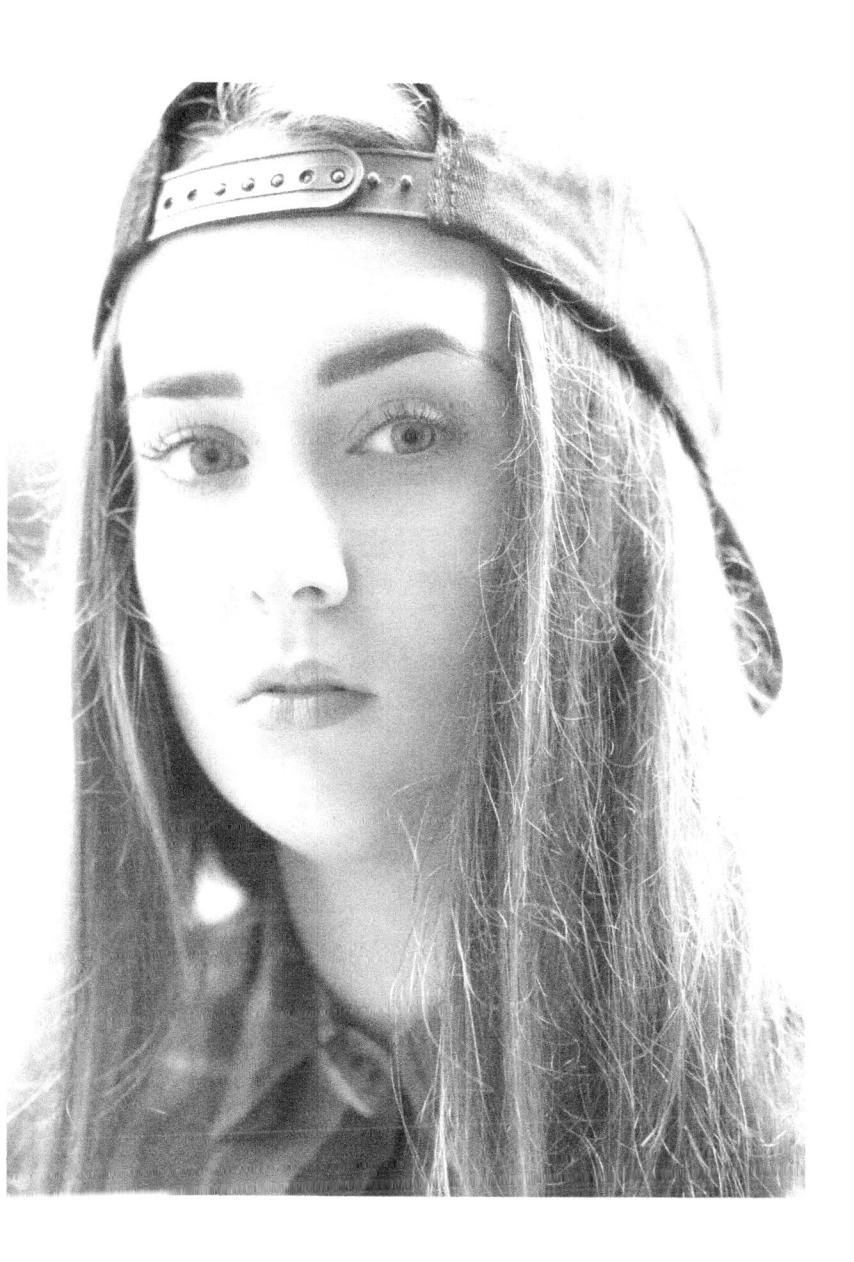

LOOK AT MY FACE!

What color are my eyes? Color my eyes.	Trace my face! I am using a: _ Black Pen _ Colored Pencil _ Marker _ Gel Pen _ Crayon _ #2 Pencil	Write one word to describe me:

COLOR THE FACES THAT SHOW HOW I FEEL:

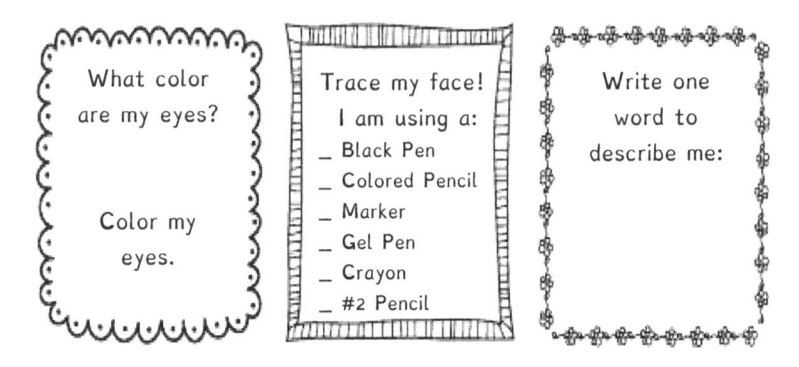

Draw me

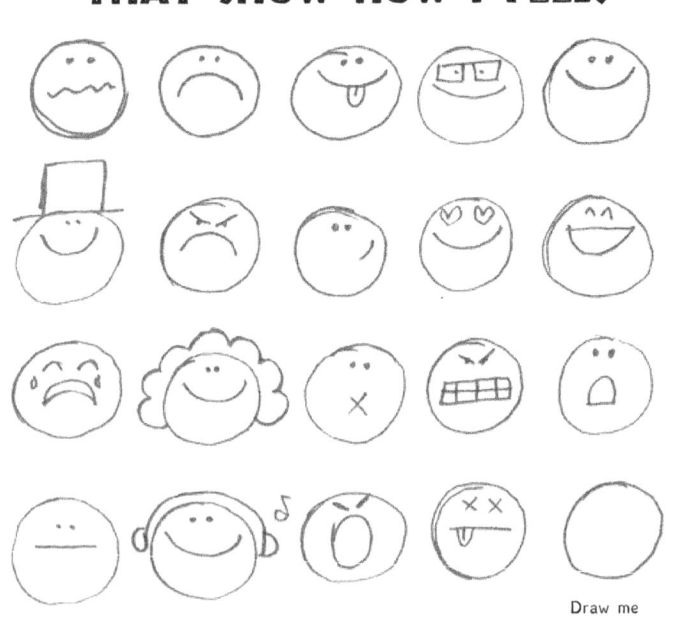

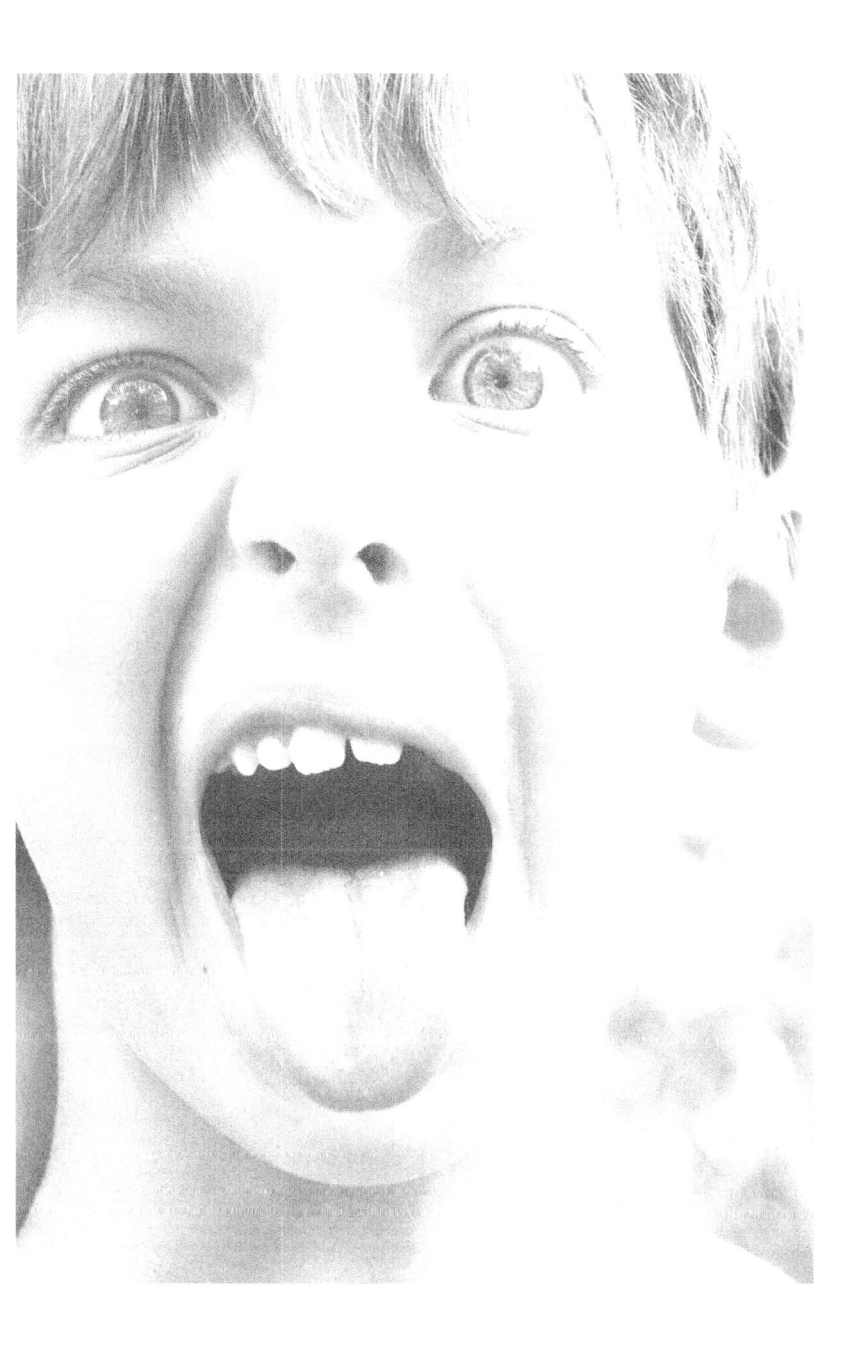

LOOK AT MY FACE!

What color are my eyes?

Color my eyes.

Trace my face!
I am using a:
- _ Black Pen
- _ Colored Pencil
- _ Marker
- _ Gel Pen
- _ Crayon
- _ #2 Pencil

Write one word to describe me:

COLOR THE FACES THAT SHOW HOW I FEEL:

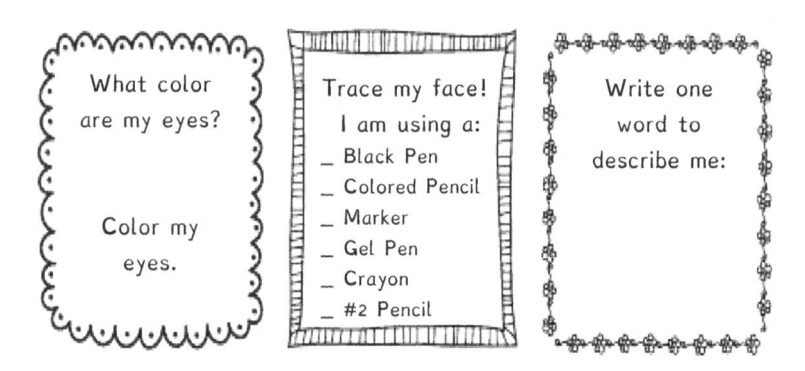

Draw me

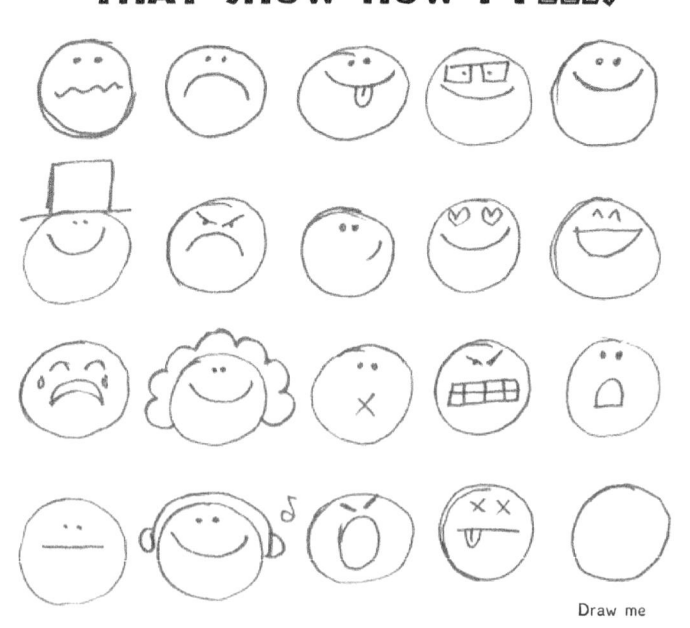

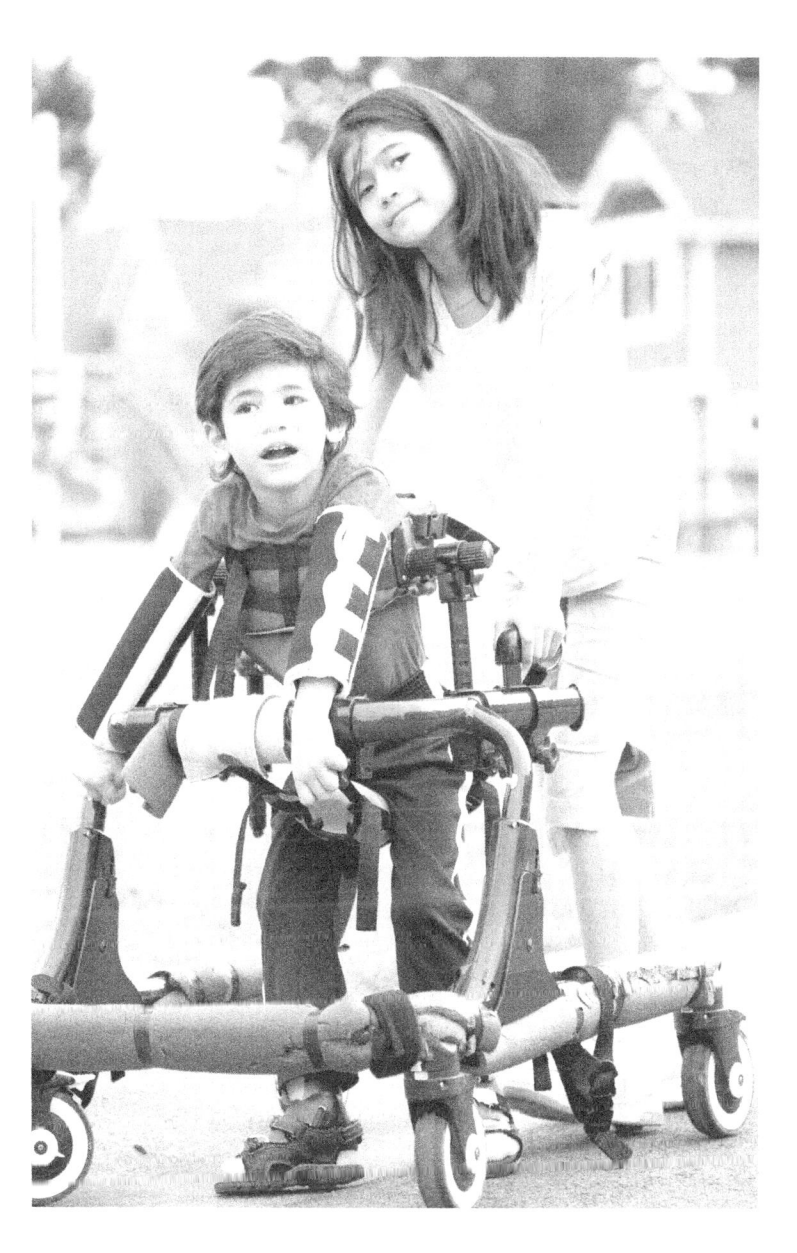

LOOK AT MY FACE!

What color are my eyes?

Color my eyes.

Trace my face!
I am using a:
_ Black Pen
_ Colored Pencil
_ Marker
_ Gel Pen
_ Crayon
_ #2 Pencil

Write one word to describe me:

COLOR THE FACES THAT SHOW HOW I FEEL:

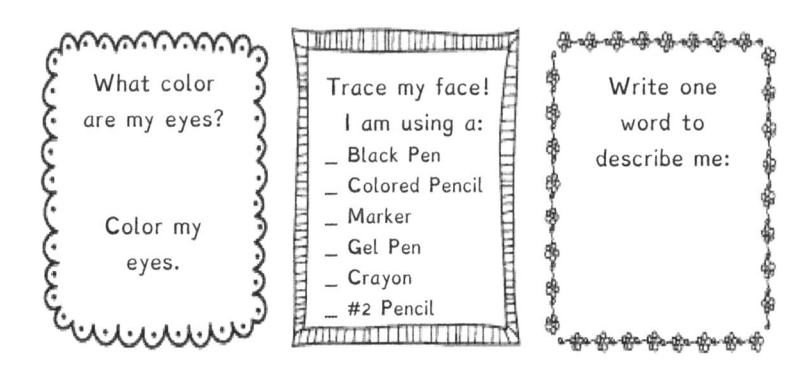

Draw me

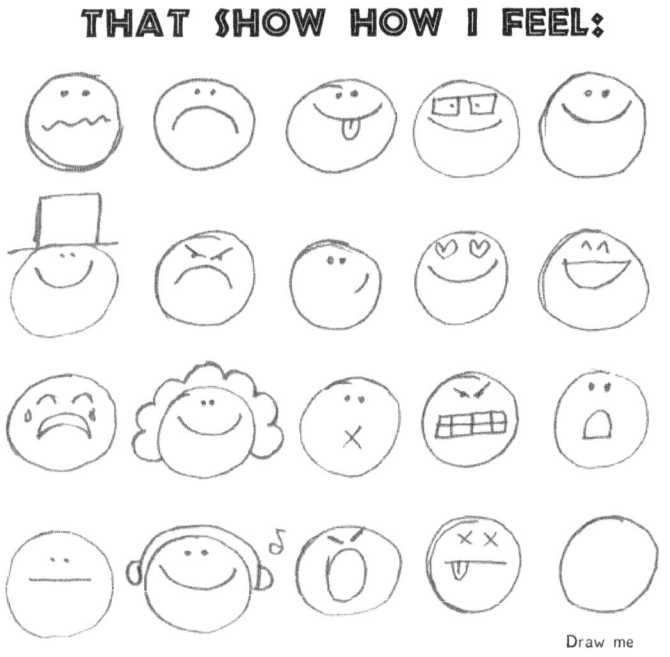

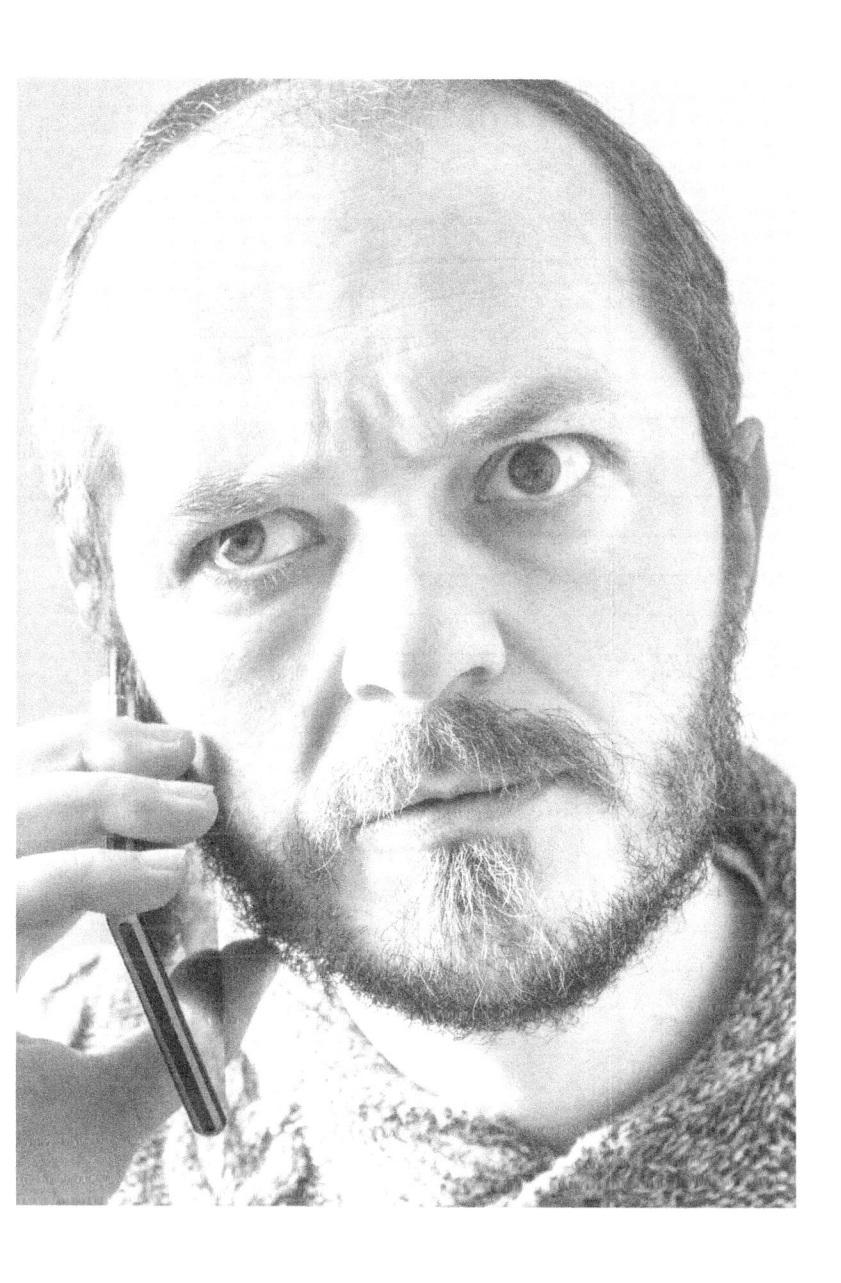

Today I am thinking about:

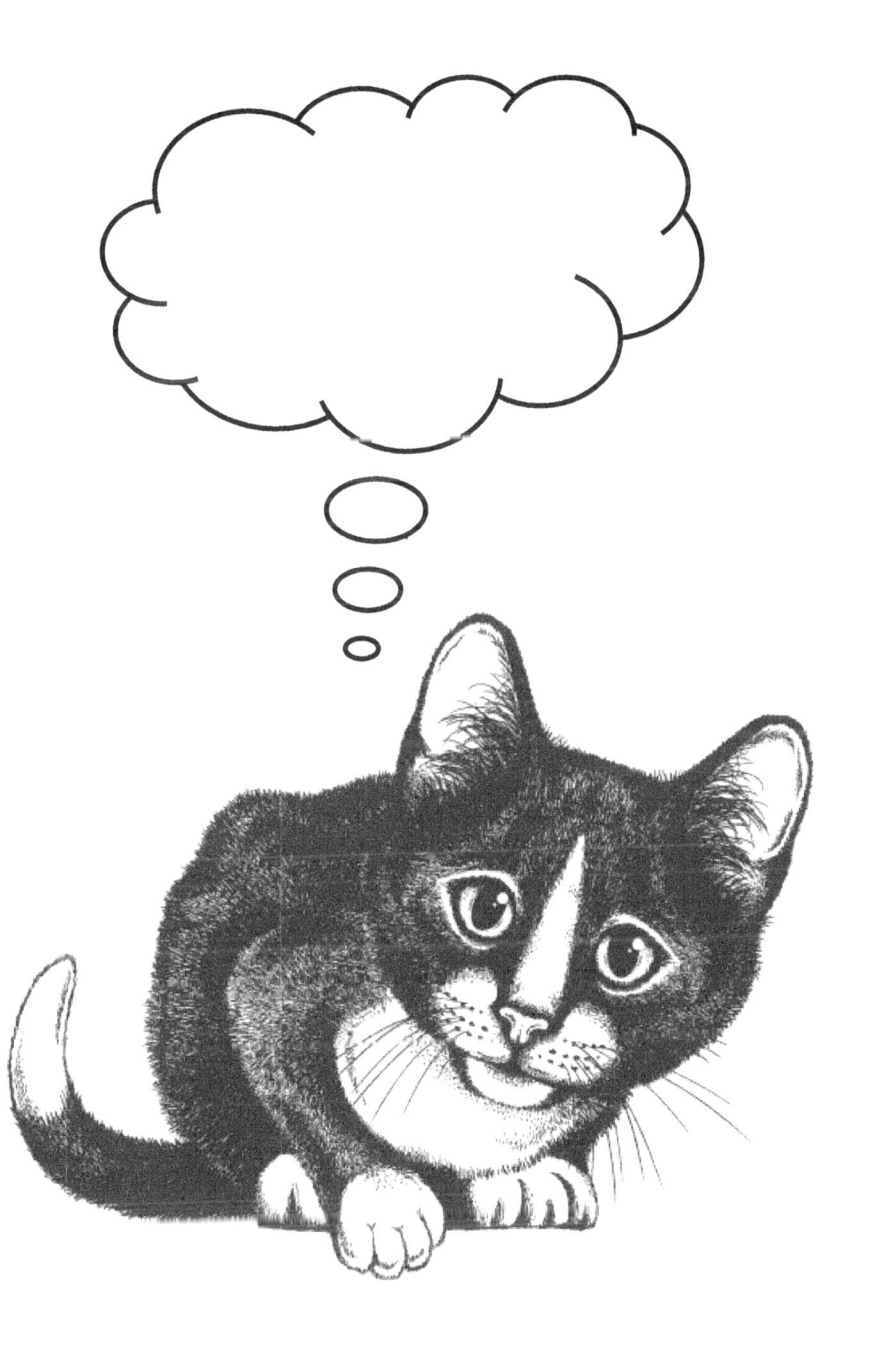

DRAW ANYTHING

LOGIC GAMES

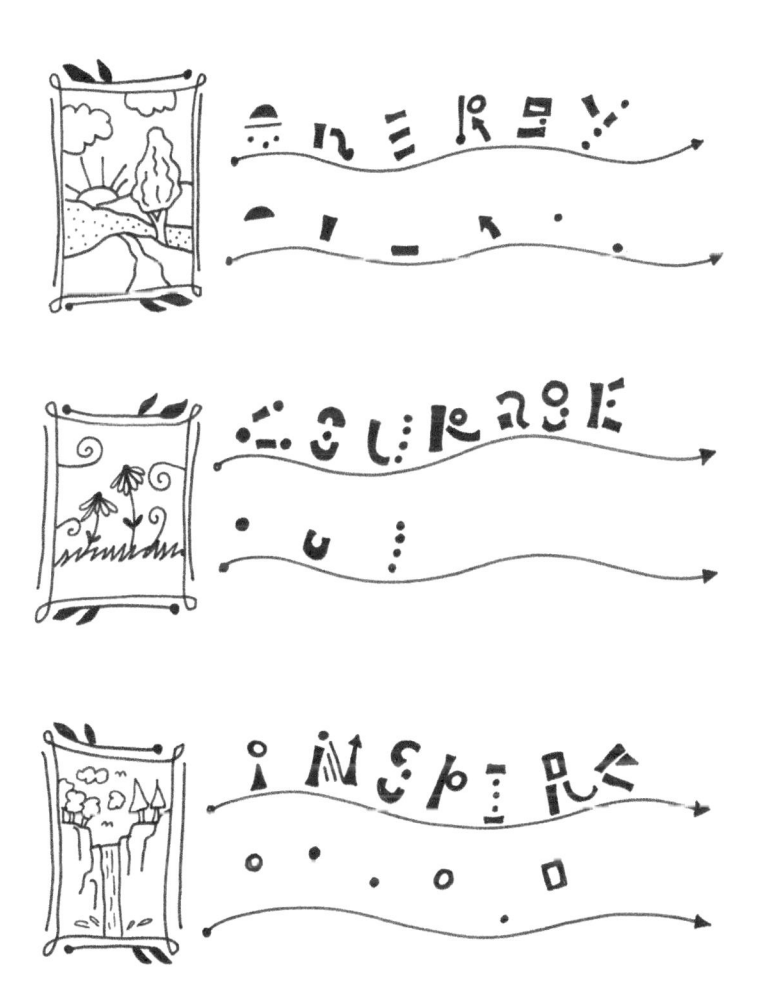

ENERGY

COURAGE

INSPIRE

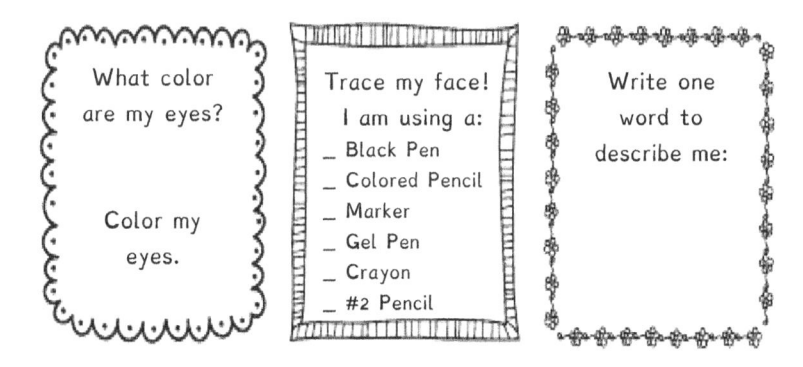

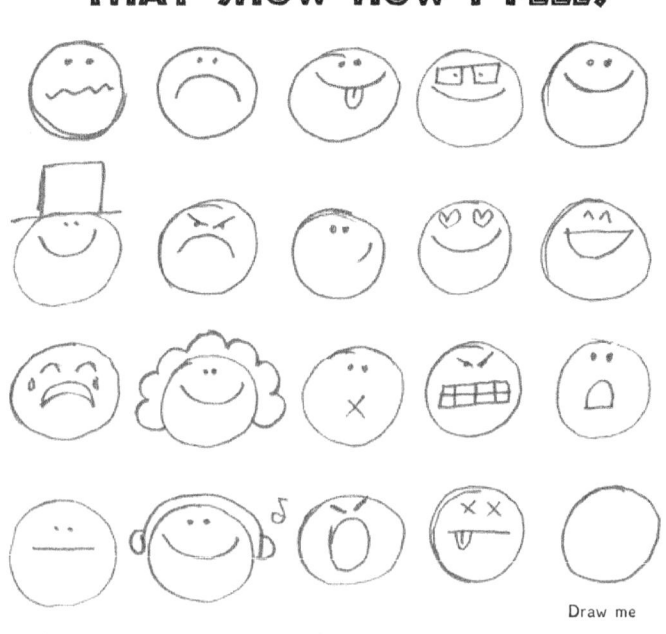

LOOK AT MY FACE!

What color are my eyes?

Color my eyes.

Trace my face!
I am using a:
- Black Pen
- Colored Pencil
- Marker
- Gel Pen
- Crayon
- #2 Pencil

Write one word to describe me:

COLOR THE FACES THAT SHOW HOW I FEEL:

Draw me

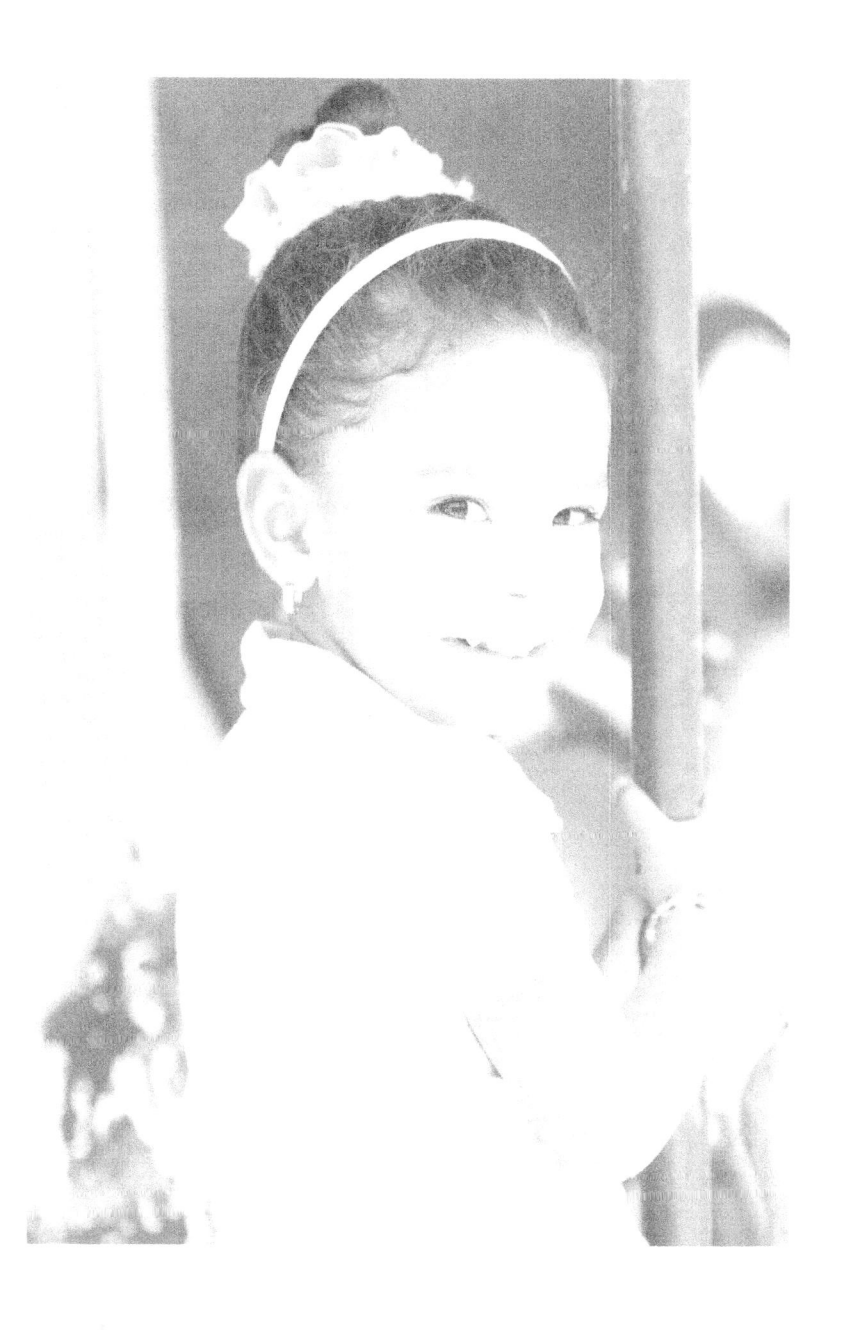

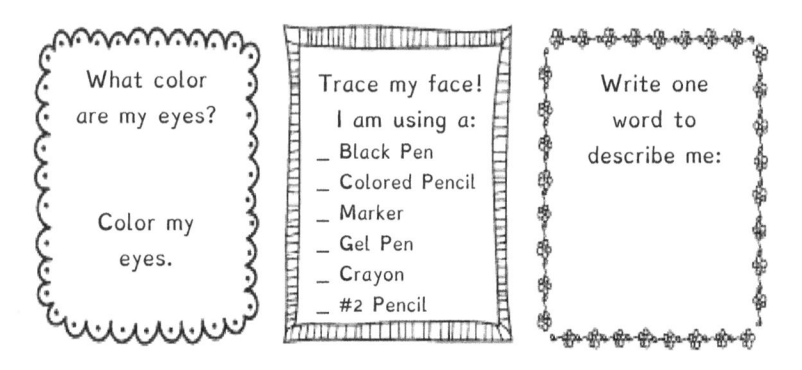

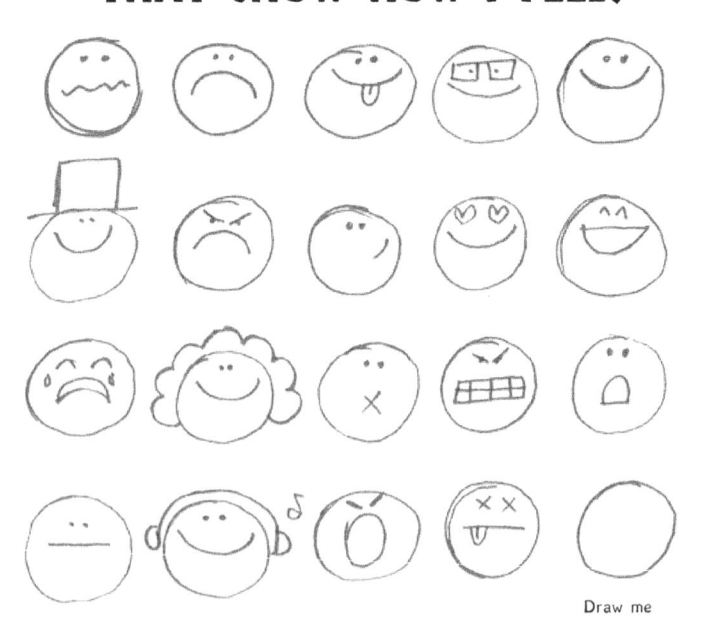

LOOK AT MY FACE!

What color are my eyes?

Color my eyes.

Trace my face! I am using a:
- _ Black Pen
- _ Colored Pencil
- _ Marker
- _ Gel Pen
- _ Crayon
- _ #2 Pencil

Write one word to describe me:

COLOR THE FACES THAT SHOW HOW I FEEL:

Draw me

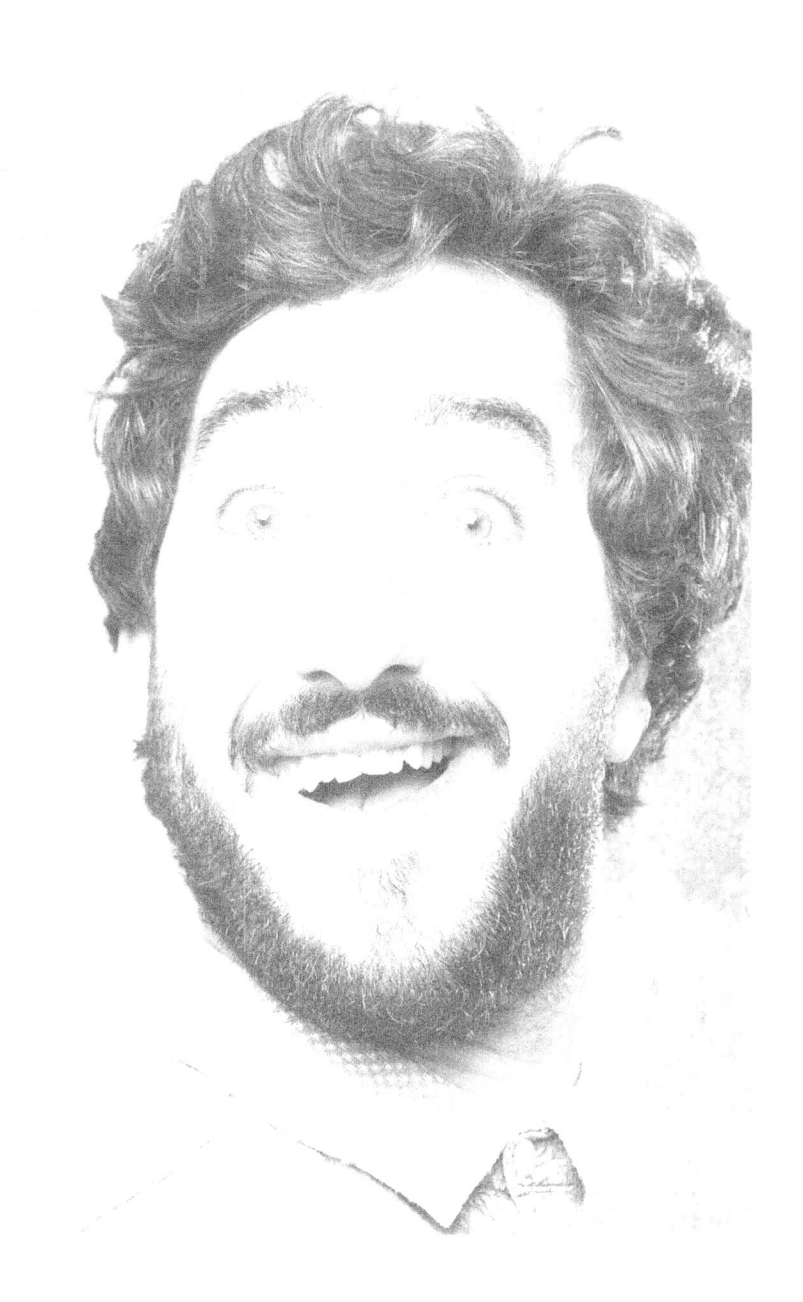

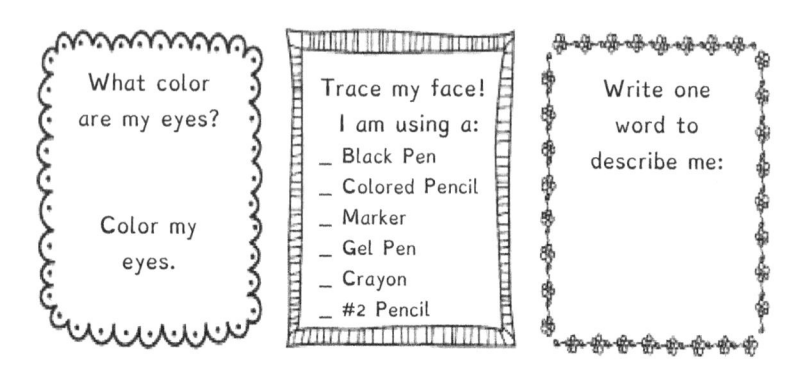

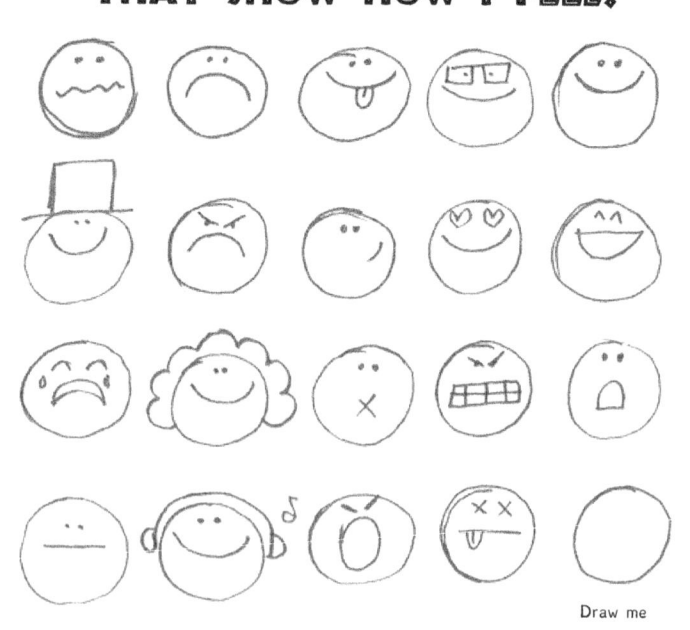

LOOK AT MY FACE!

What color are my eyes?

Color my eyes.

Trace my face!
I am using a:
- Black Pen
- Colored Pencil
- Marker
- Gel Pen
- Crayon
- #2 Pencil

Write one word to describe me:

COLOR THE FACES THAT SHOW HOW I FEEL:

Draw me

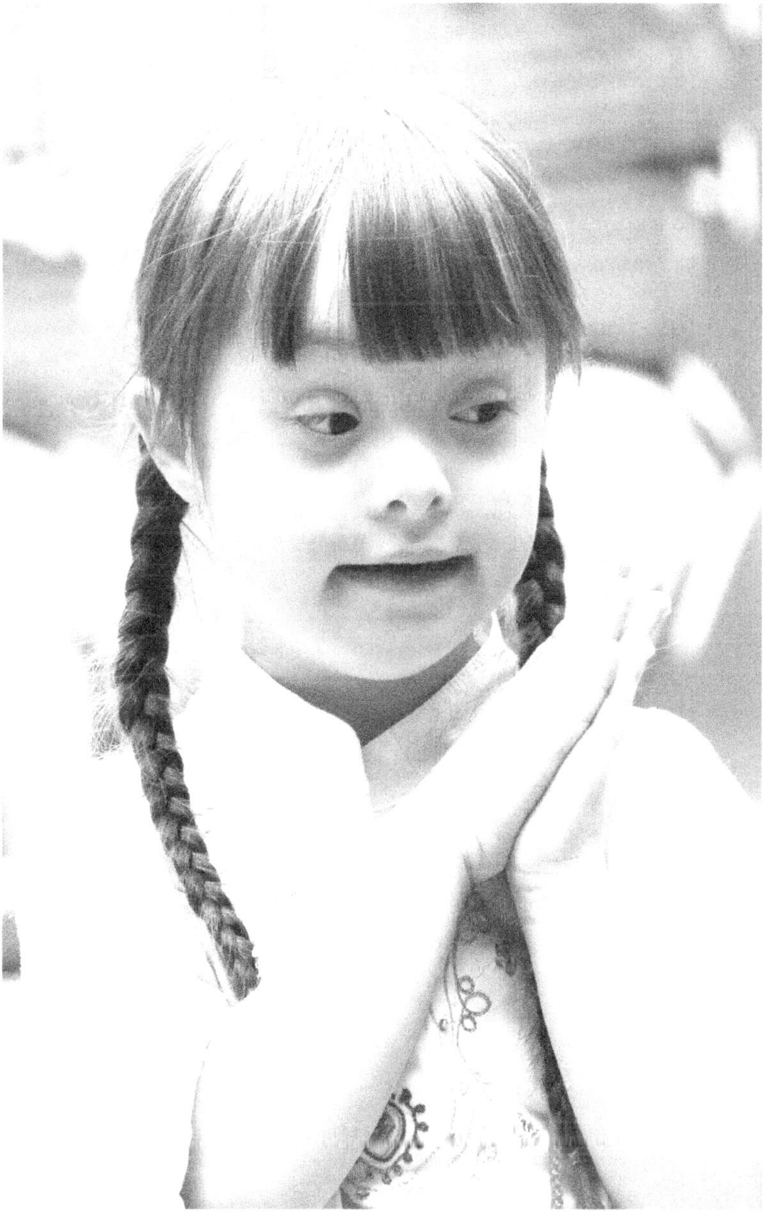

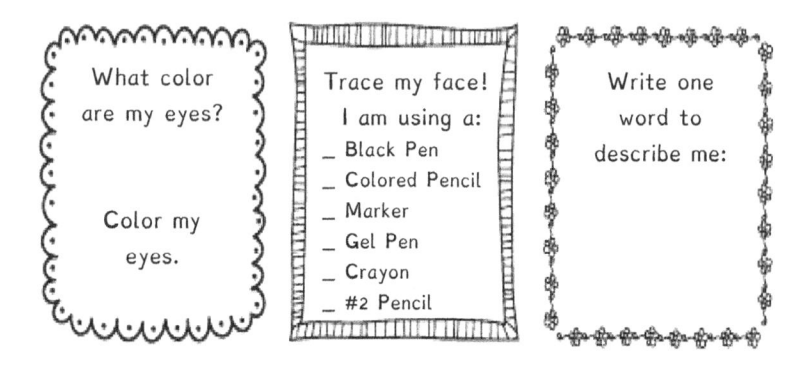

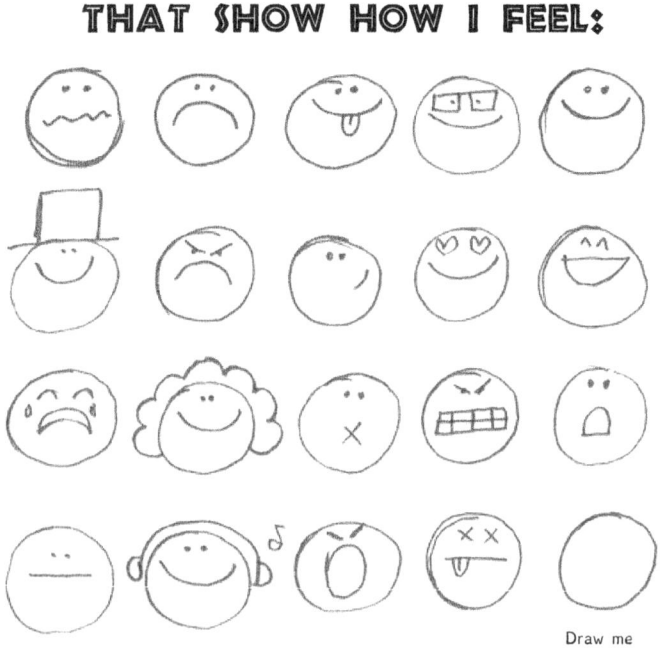

LOOK AT MY FACE!

What color are my eyes?

Color my eyes.

Trace my face!
I am using a:
- Black Pen
- Colored Pencil
- Marker
- Gel Pen
- Crayon
- #2 Pencil

Write one word to describe me:

COLOR THE FACES THAT SHOW HOW I FEEL:

Draw me

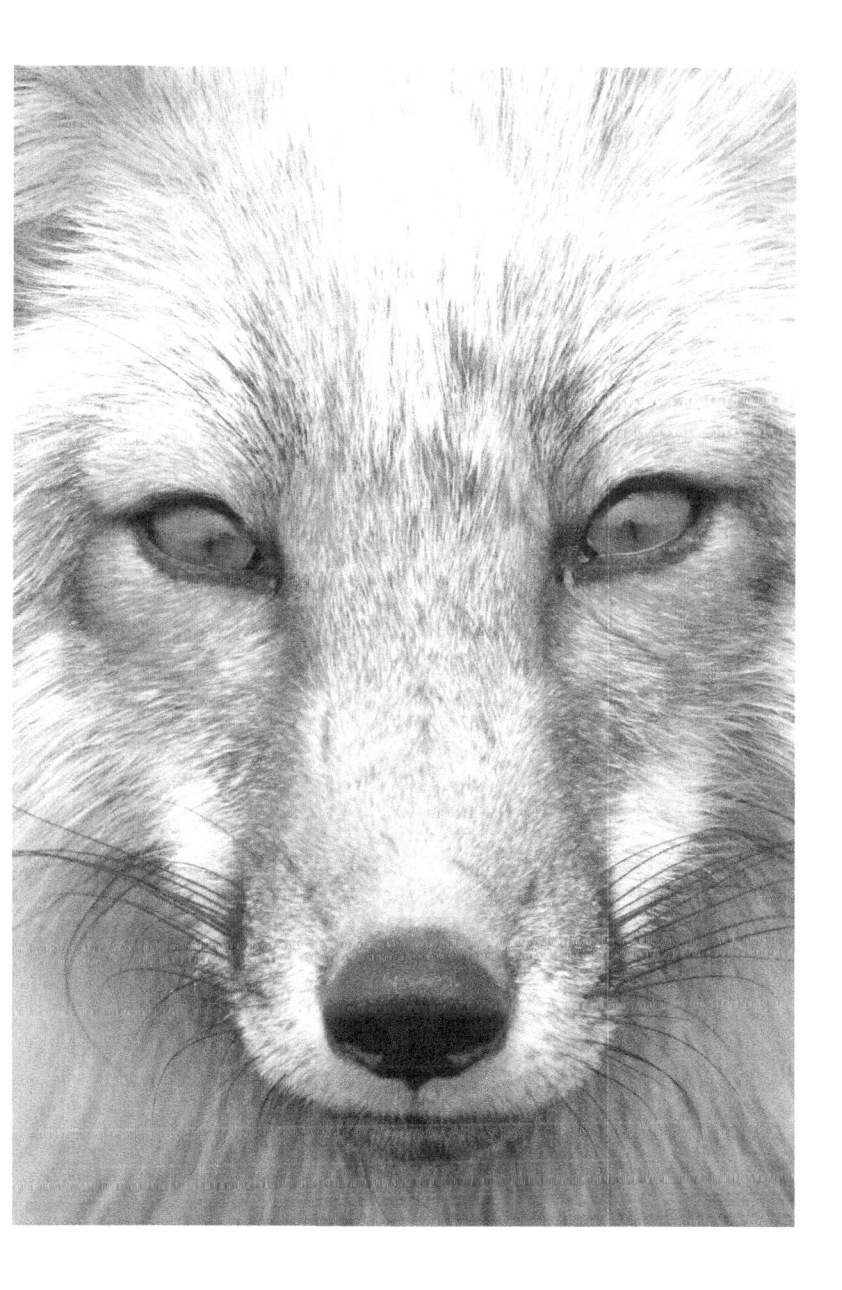

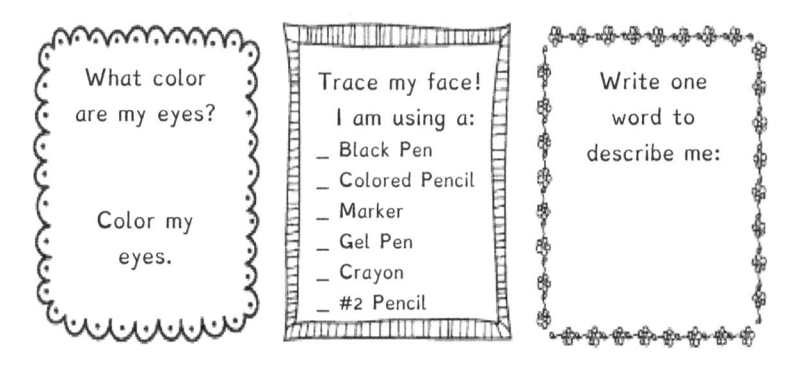

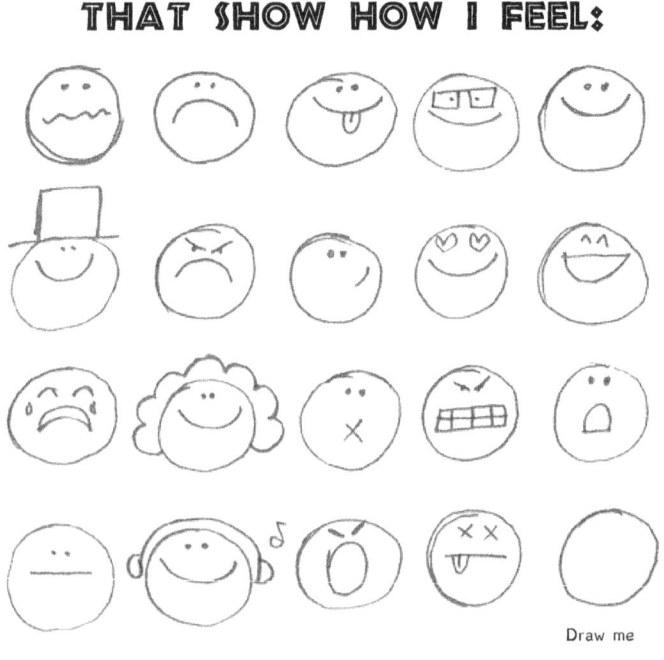

LOOK AT MY FACE!

| What color are my eyes? Color my eyes. | Trace my face! I am using a: _ Black Pen _ Colored Pencil _ Marker _ Gel Pen _ Crayon _ #2 Pencil | Write one word to describe me: |

COLOR THE FACES THAT SHOW HOW I FEEL:

Draw me

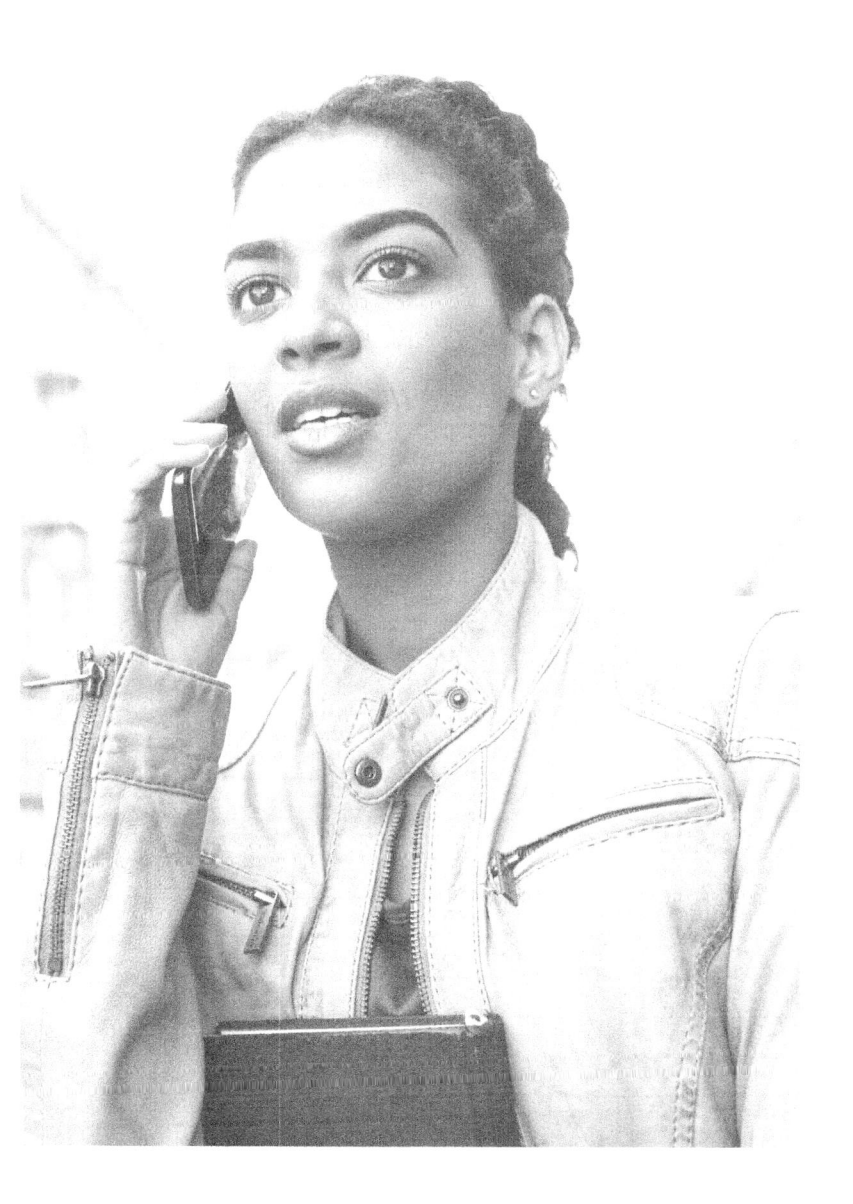

Today I am thinking about:

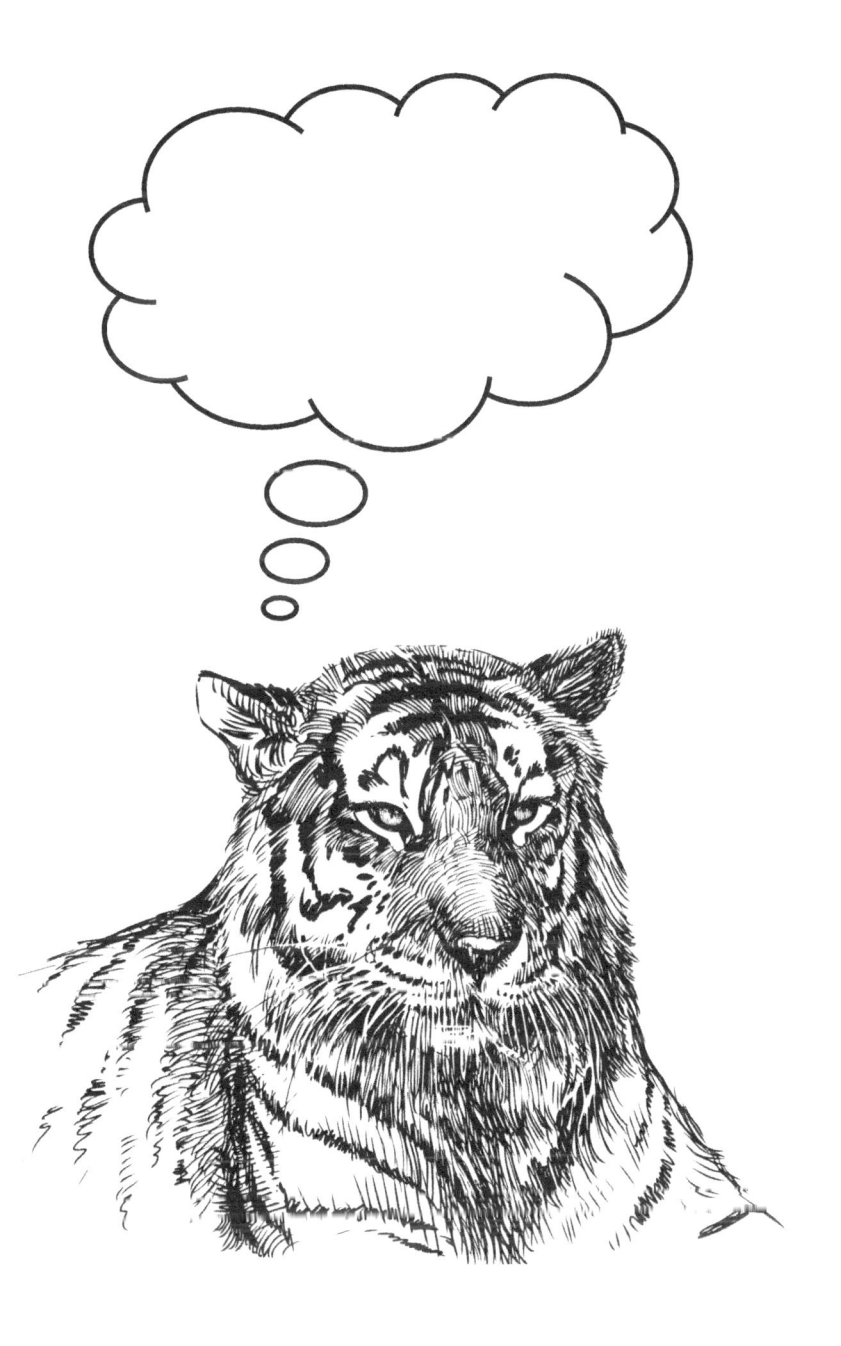

DRAW ANYTHING

LOGIC GAMES

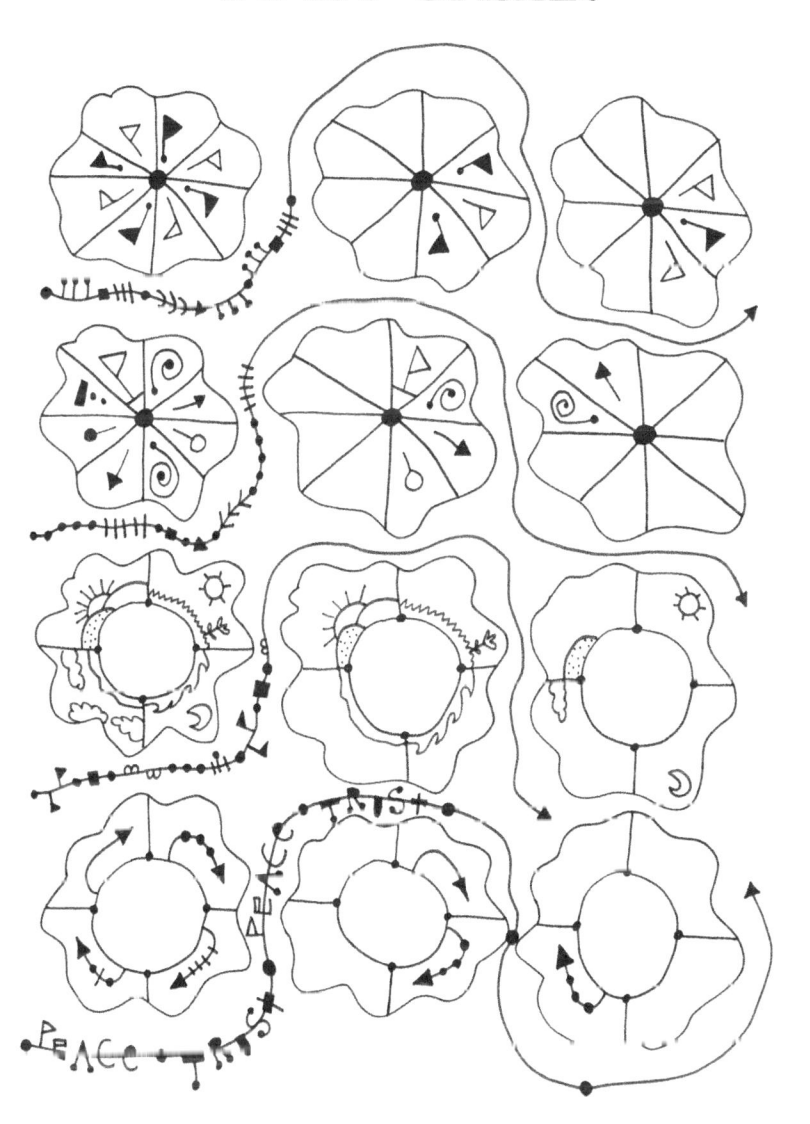

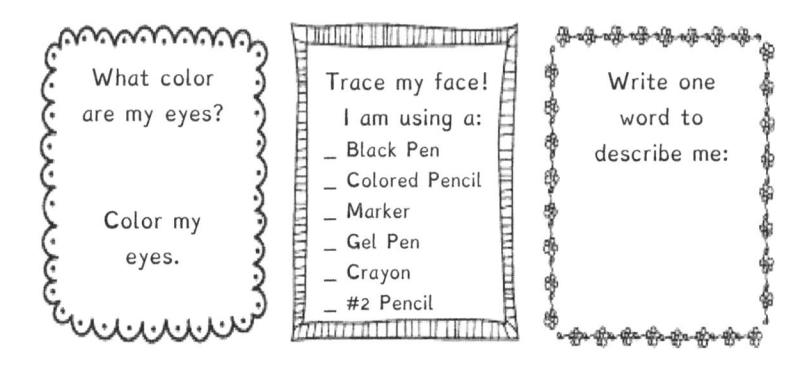

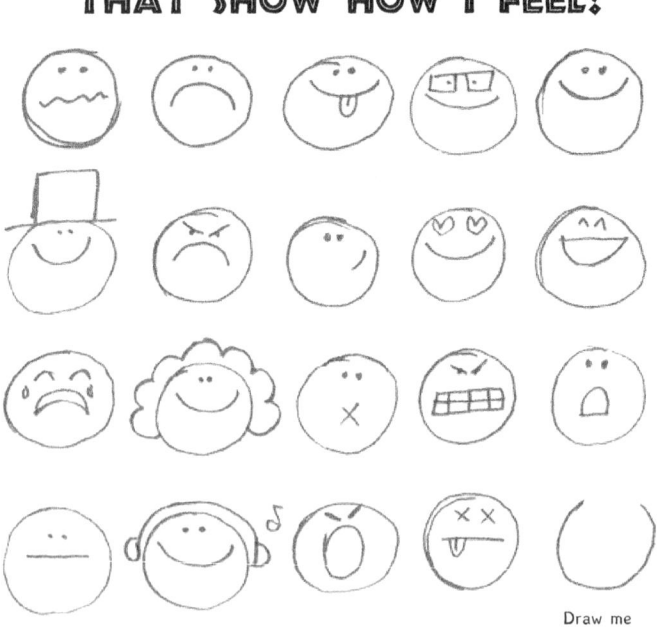

LOOK AT MY FACE!

What color are my eyes?

Color my eyes.

Trace my face!
I am using a:
_ Black Pen
_ Colored Pencil
_ Marker
_ Gel Pen
_ Crayon
_ #2 Pencil

Write one word to describe me:

COLOR THE FACES THAT SHOW HOW I FEEL:

Draw me

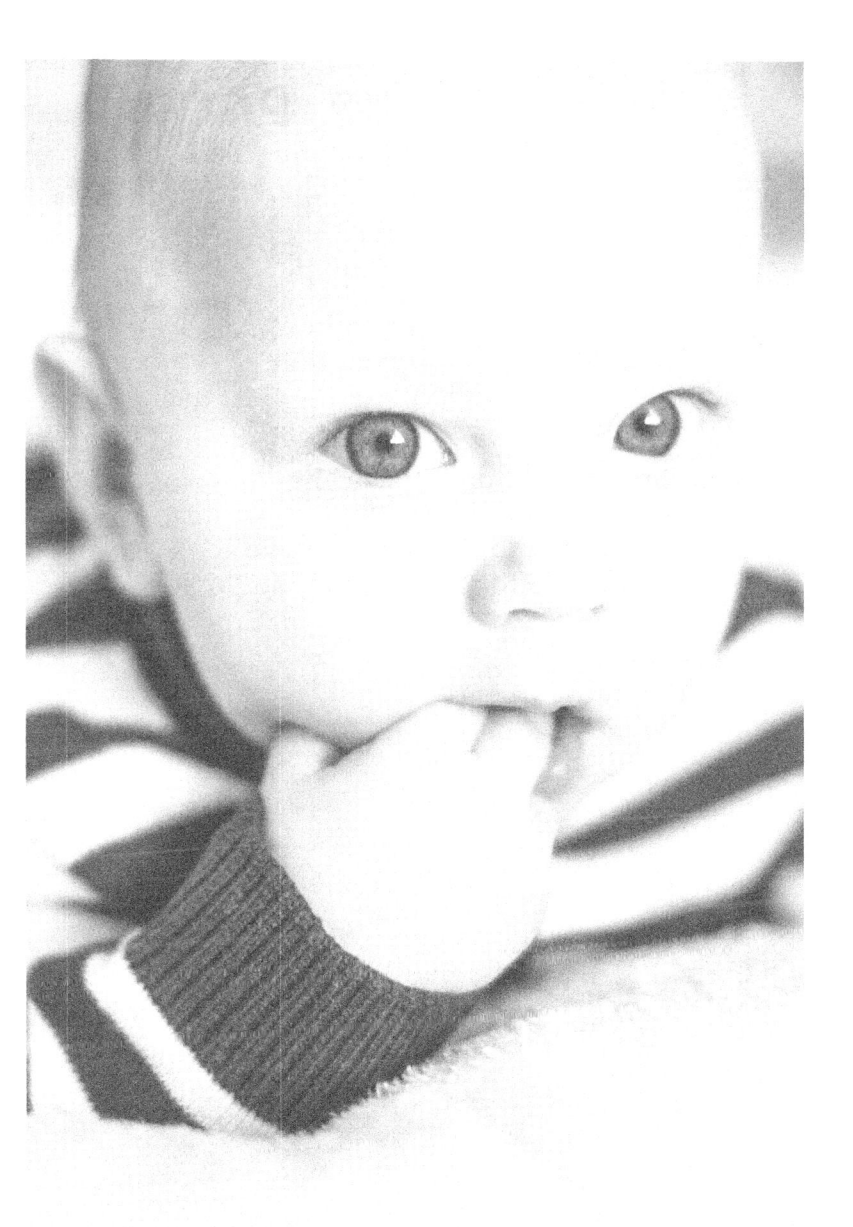

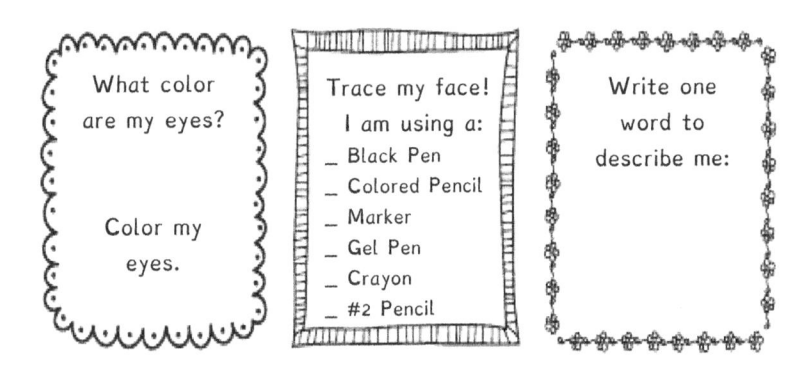

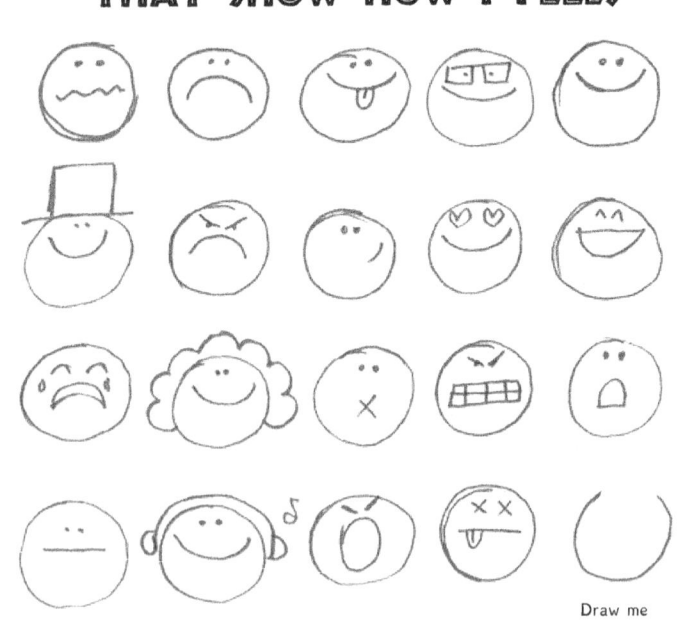

LOOK AT MY FACE!

| What color are my eyes? Color my eyes. | Trace my face! I am using a: _ Black Pen _ Colored Pencil _ Marker _ Gel Pen _ Crayon _ #2 Pencil | Write one word to describe me: |

COLOR THE FACES THAT SHOW HOW I FEEL:

Draw me

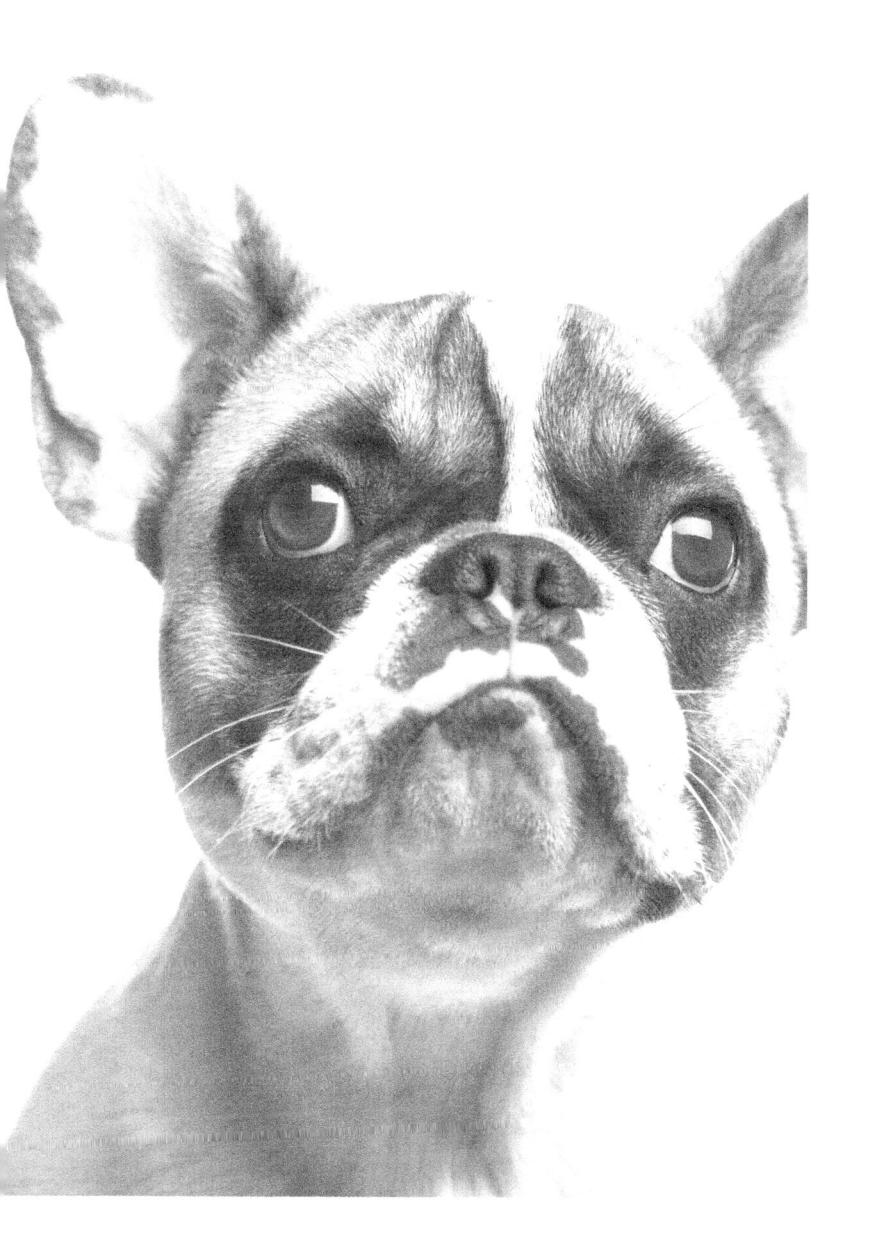

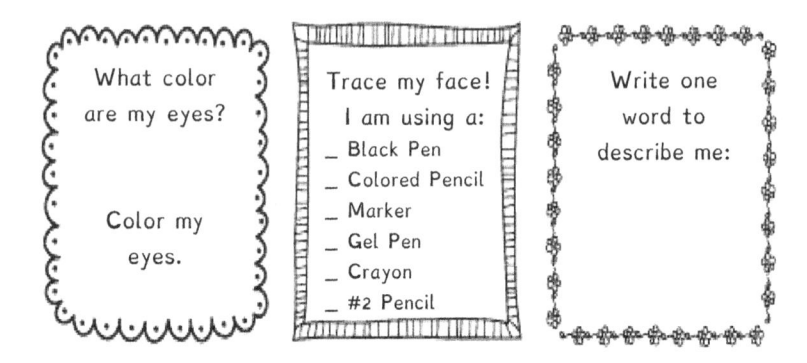

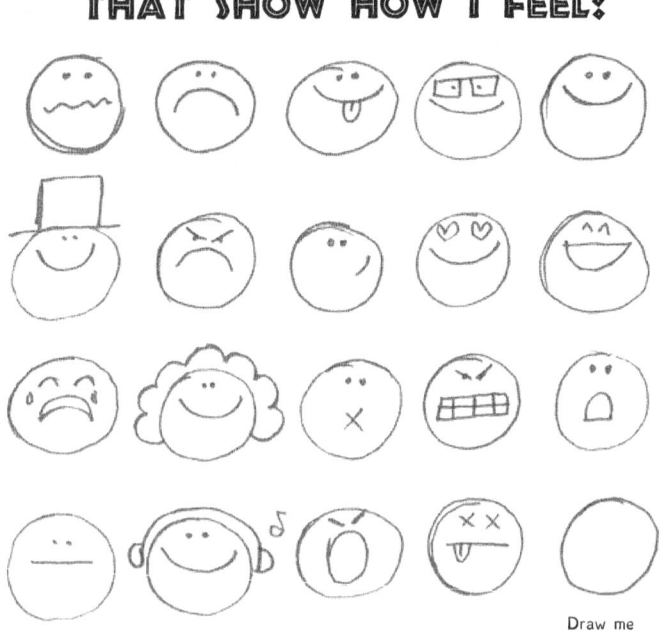

LOOK AT MY FACE!

What color are my eyes?

Color my eyes.

Trace my face!
I am using a:
_ Black Pen
_ Colored Pencil
_ Marker
_ Gel Pen
_ Crayon
_ #2 Pencil

Write one word to describe me:

COLOR THE FACES THAT SHOW HOW I FEEL:

Draw me

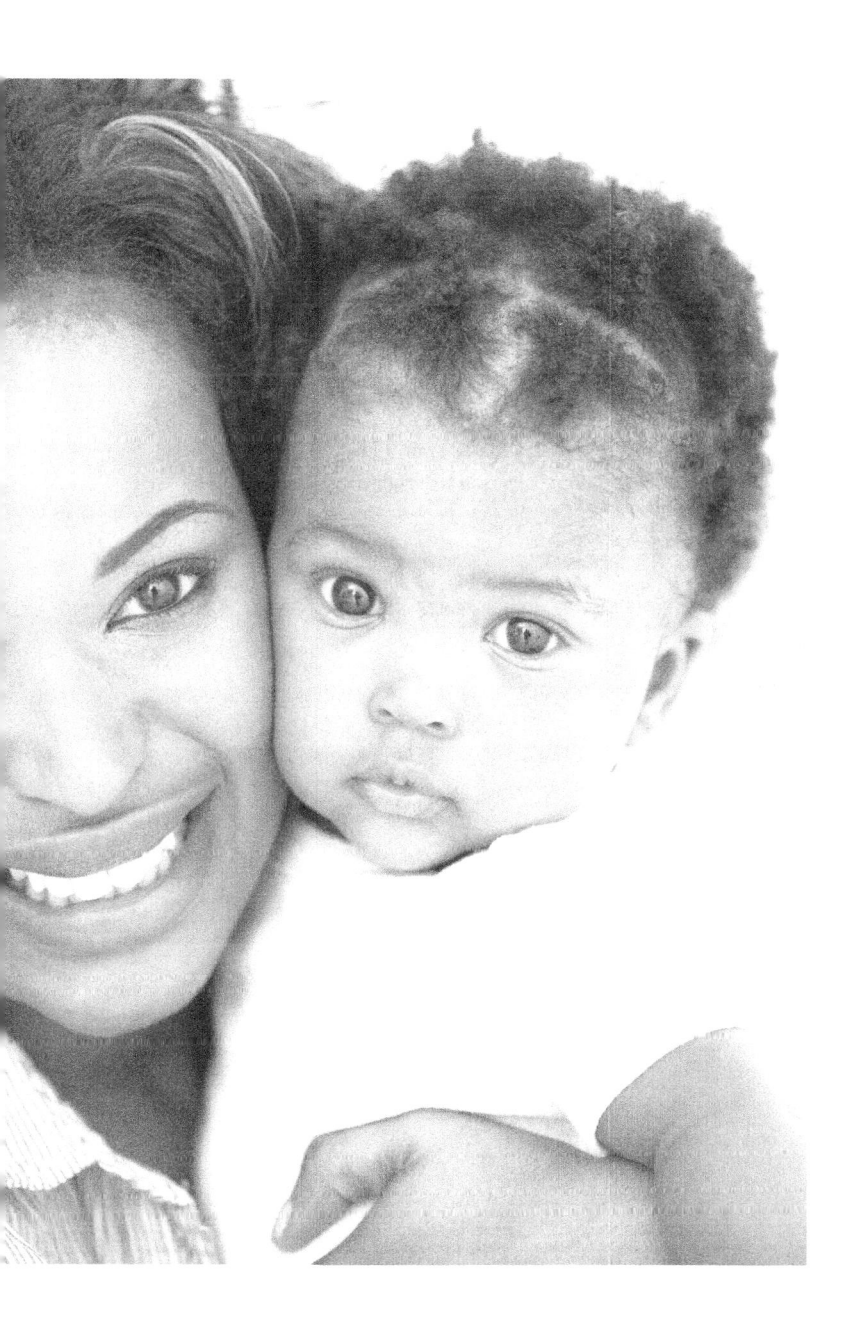

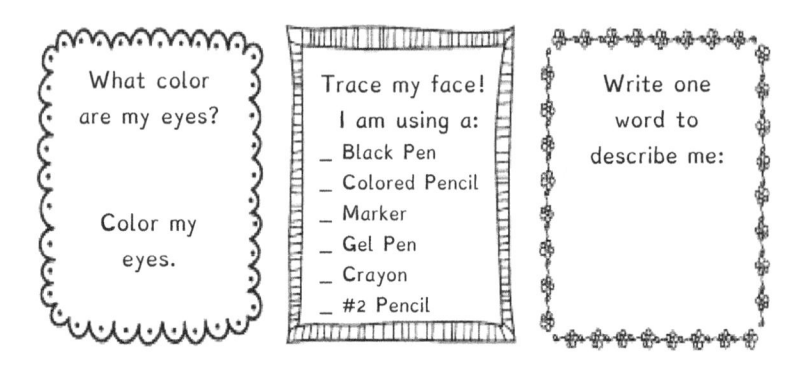

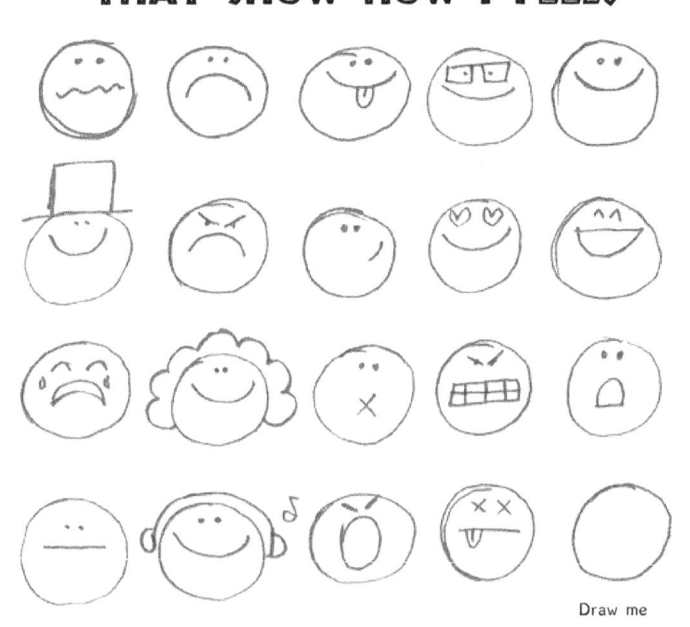

LOOK AT MY FACE!

What color are my eyes?

Color my eyes.

Trace my face!
I am using a:
- Black Pen
- Colored Pencil
- Marker
- Gel Pen
- Crayon
- #2 Pencil

Write one word to describe me:

COLOR THE FACES THAT SHOW HOW I FEEL:

Draw me

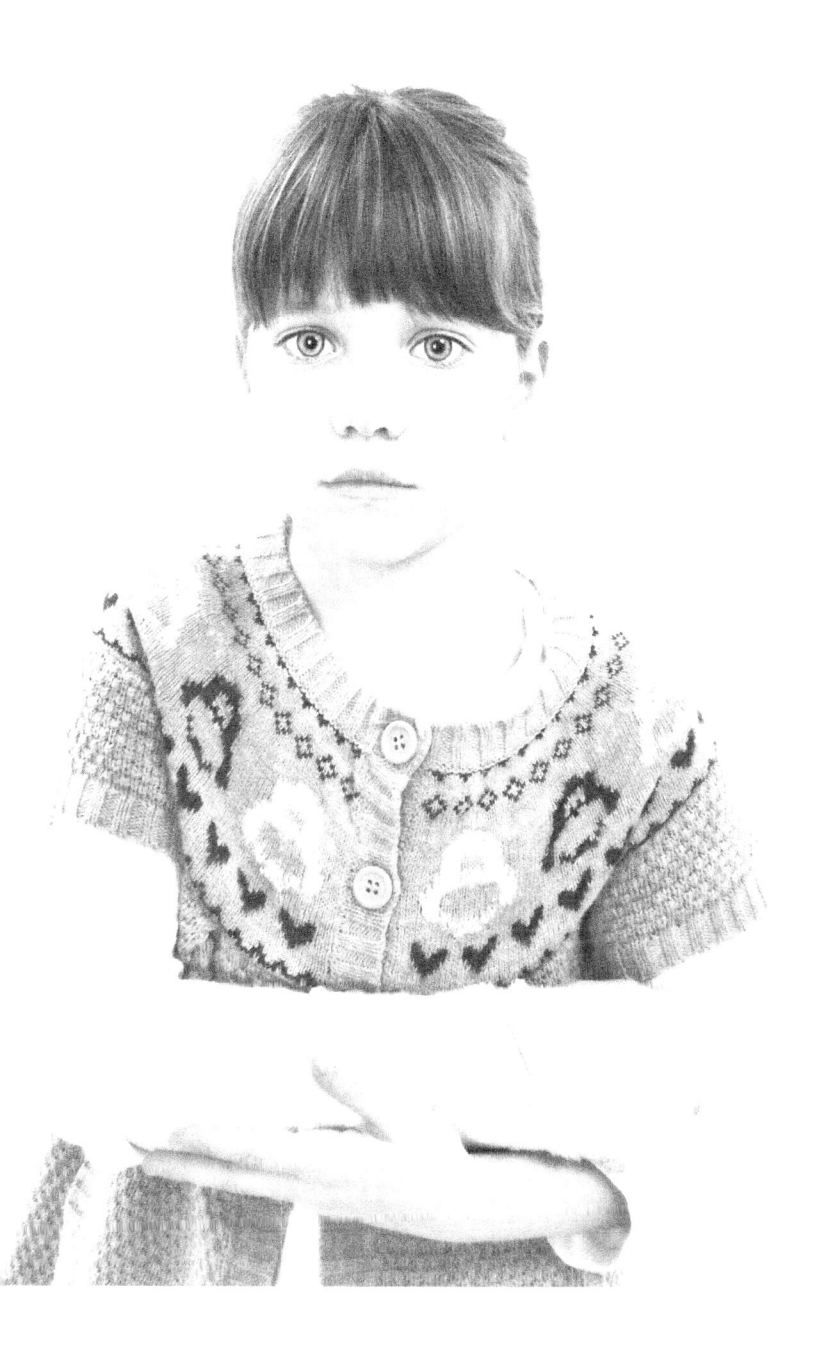

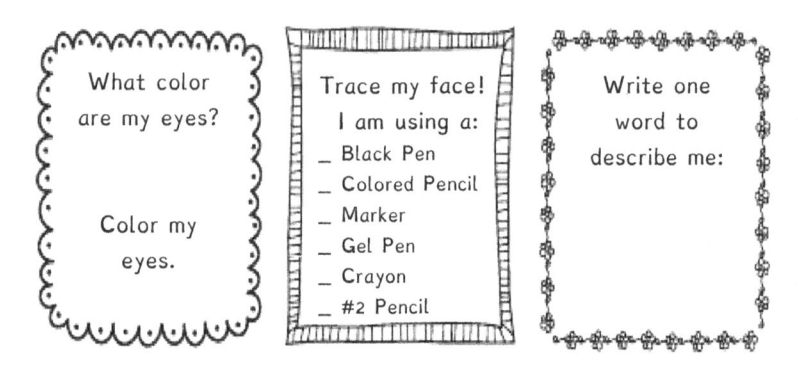

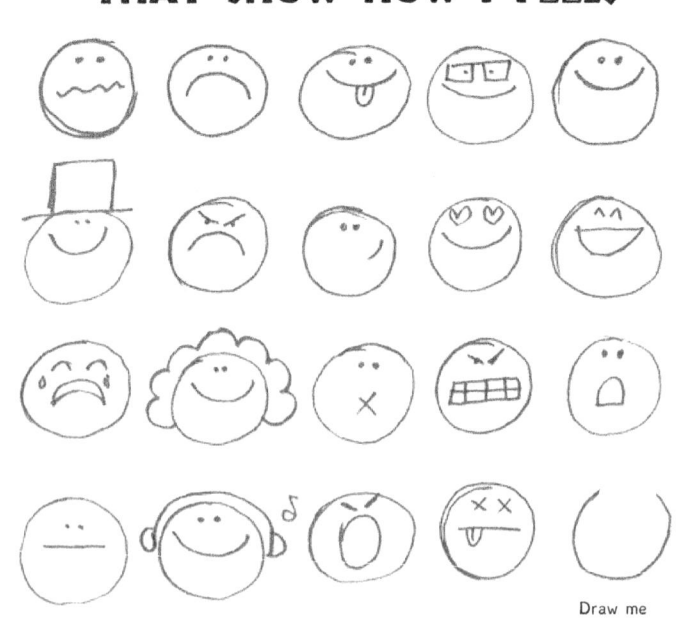

LOOK AT MY FACE!

What color are my eyes?

Color my eyes.

Trace my face! I am using a:
_ Black Pen
_ Colored Pencil
_ Marker
_ Gel Pen
_ Crayon
_ #2 Pencil

Write one word to describe me:

COLOR THE FACES THAT SHOW HOW I FEEL:

Draw me

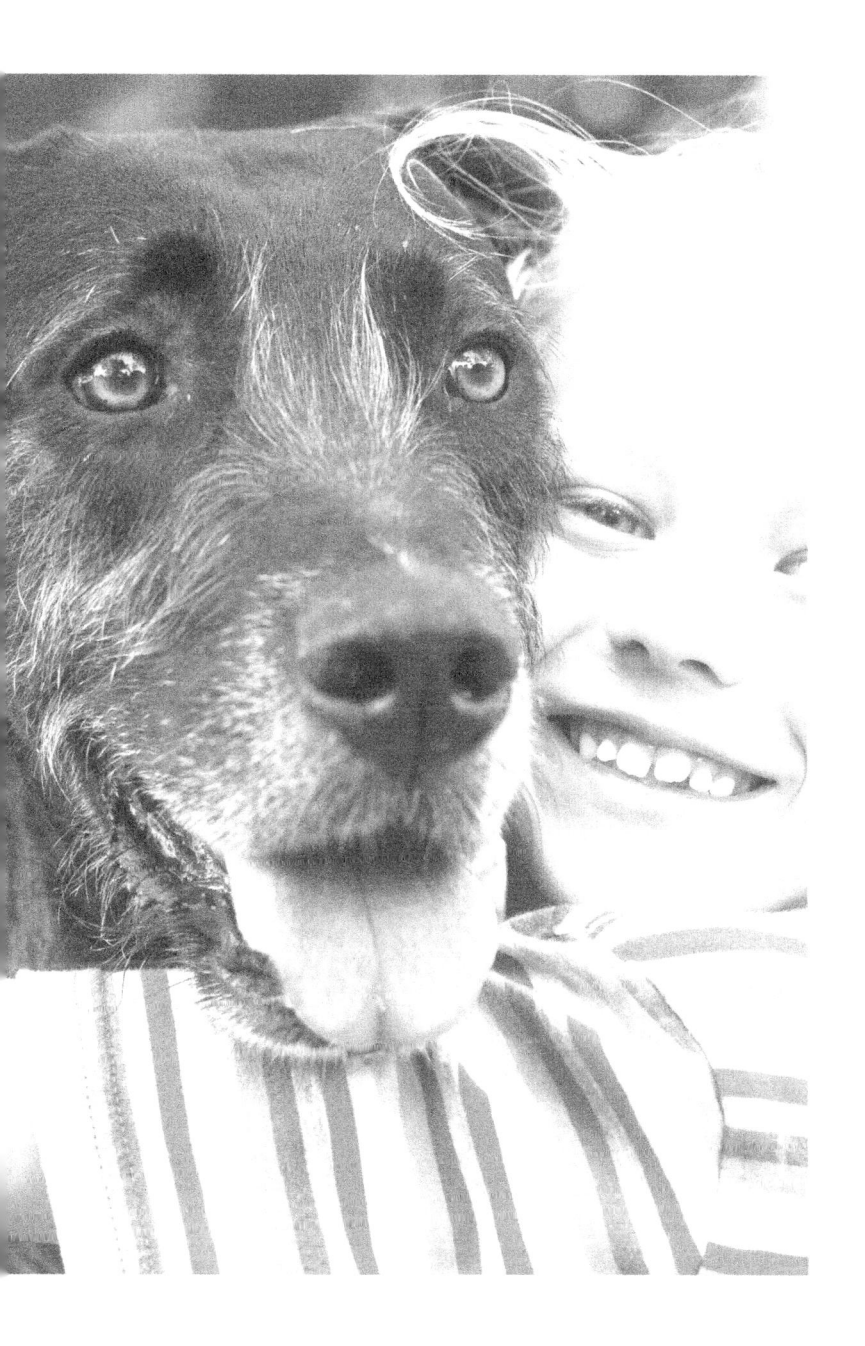

Today I am thinking about:

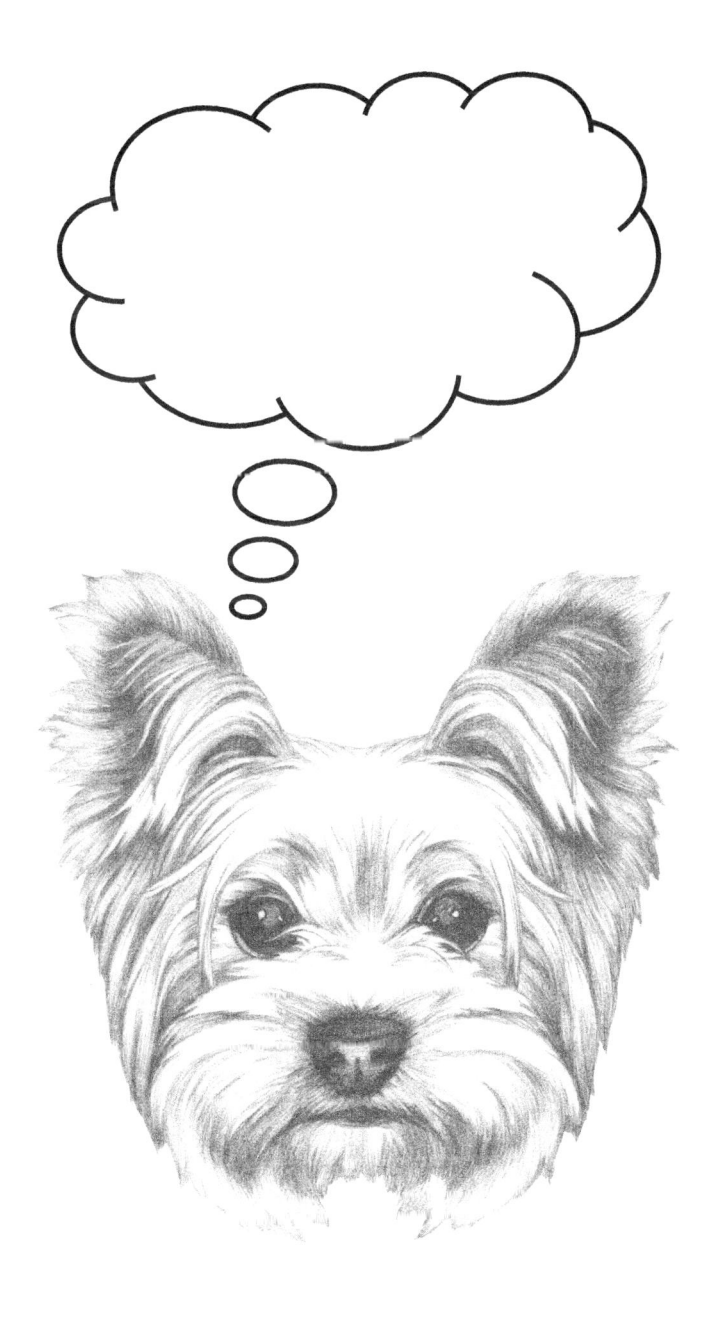

DRAW ANYTHING

LOGIC GAMES

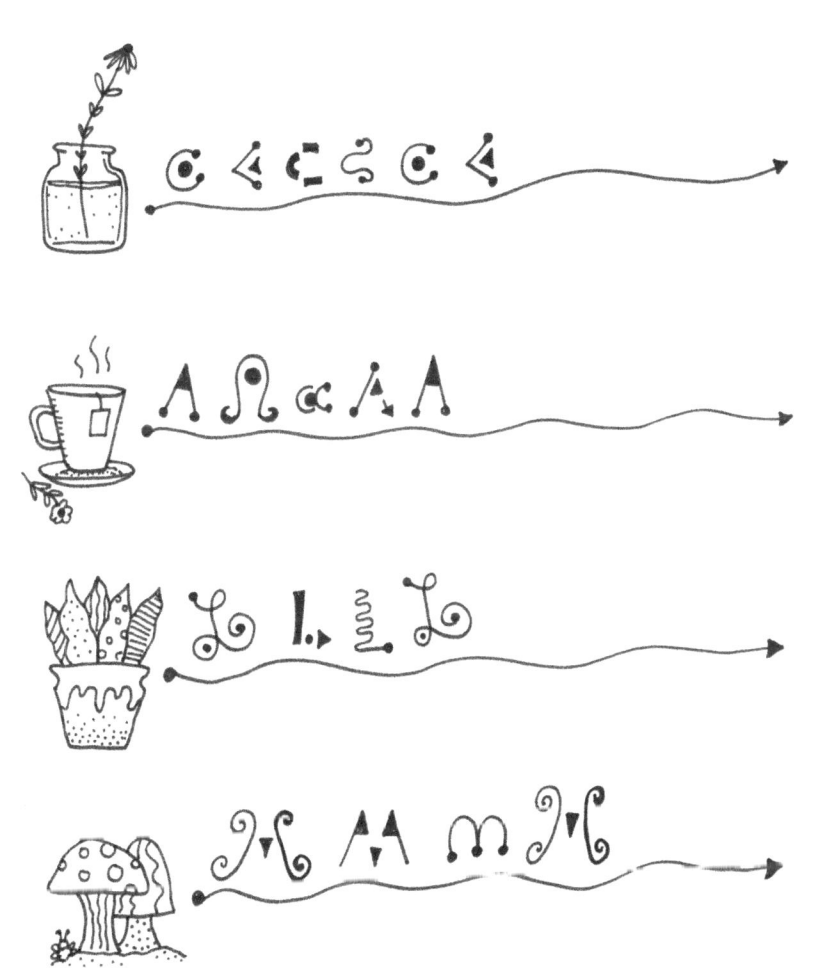

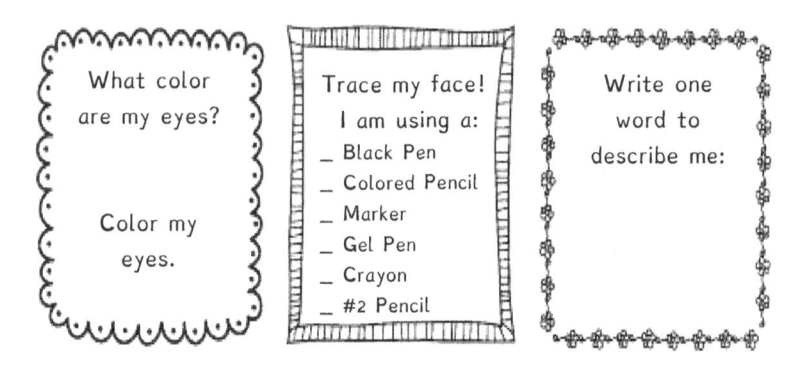

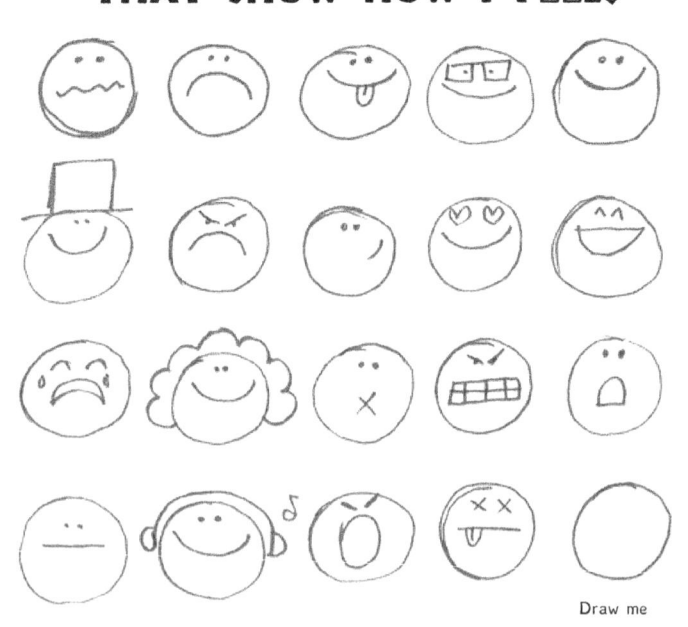

LOOK AT MY FACE!

What color are my eyes?

Color my eyes.

Trace my face!
I am using a:
_ Black Pen
_ Colored Pencil
_ Marker
_ Gel Pen
_ Crayon
_ #2 Pencil

Write one word to describe me:

COLOR THE FACES THAT SHOW HOW I FEEL:

Draw me

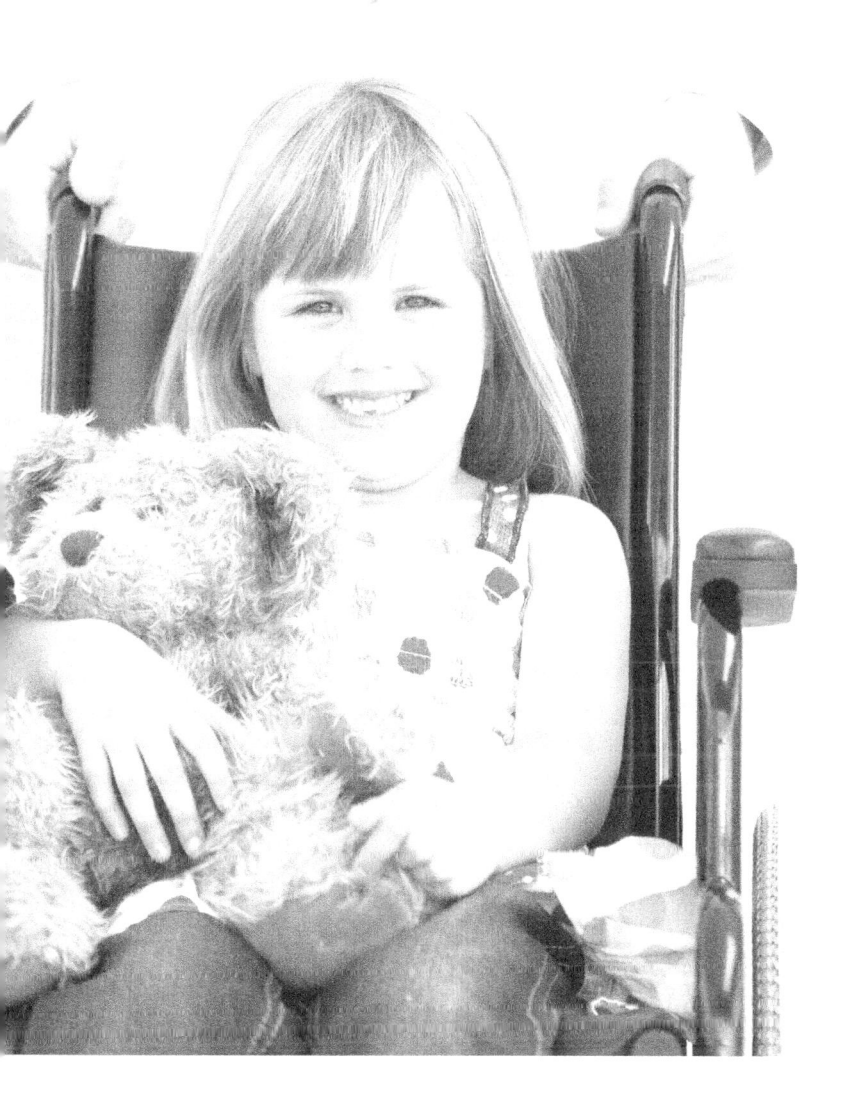

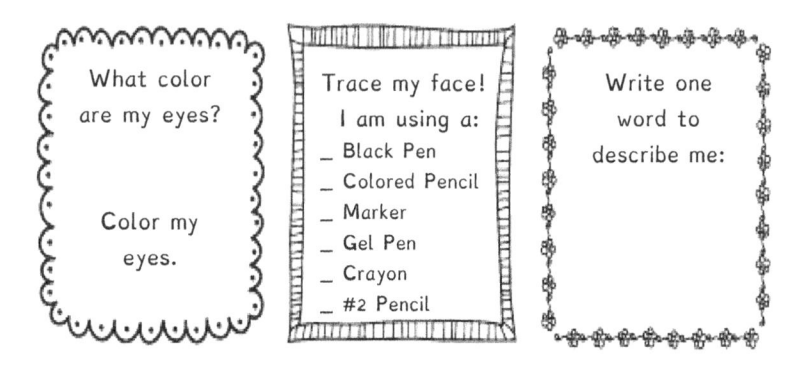

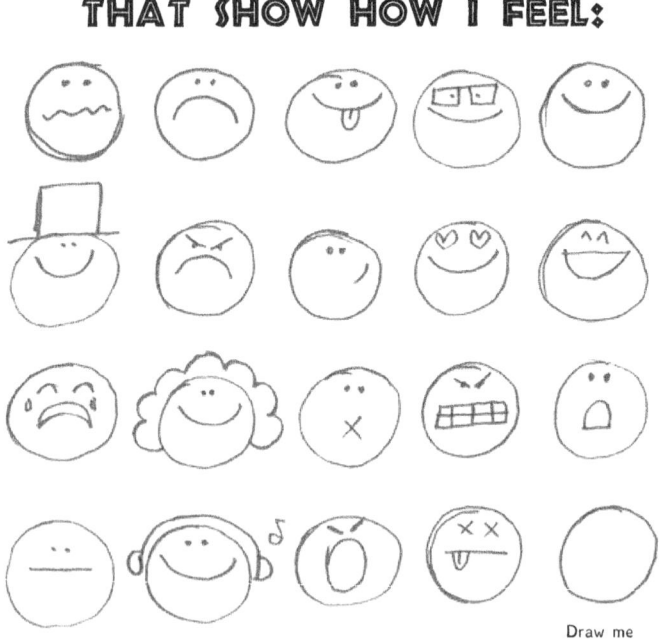

LOOK AT MY FACE!

What color are my eyes?

Color my eyes.

Trace my face!
I am using a:
_ Black Pen
_ Colored Pencil
_ Marker
_ Gel Pen
_ Crayon
_ #2 Pencil

Write one word to describe me:

COLOR THE FACES THAT SHOW HOW I FEEL:

Draw me

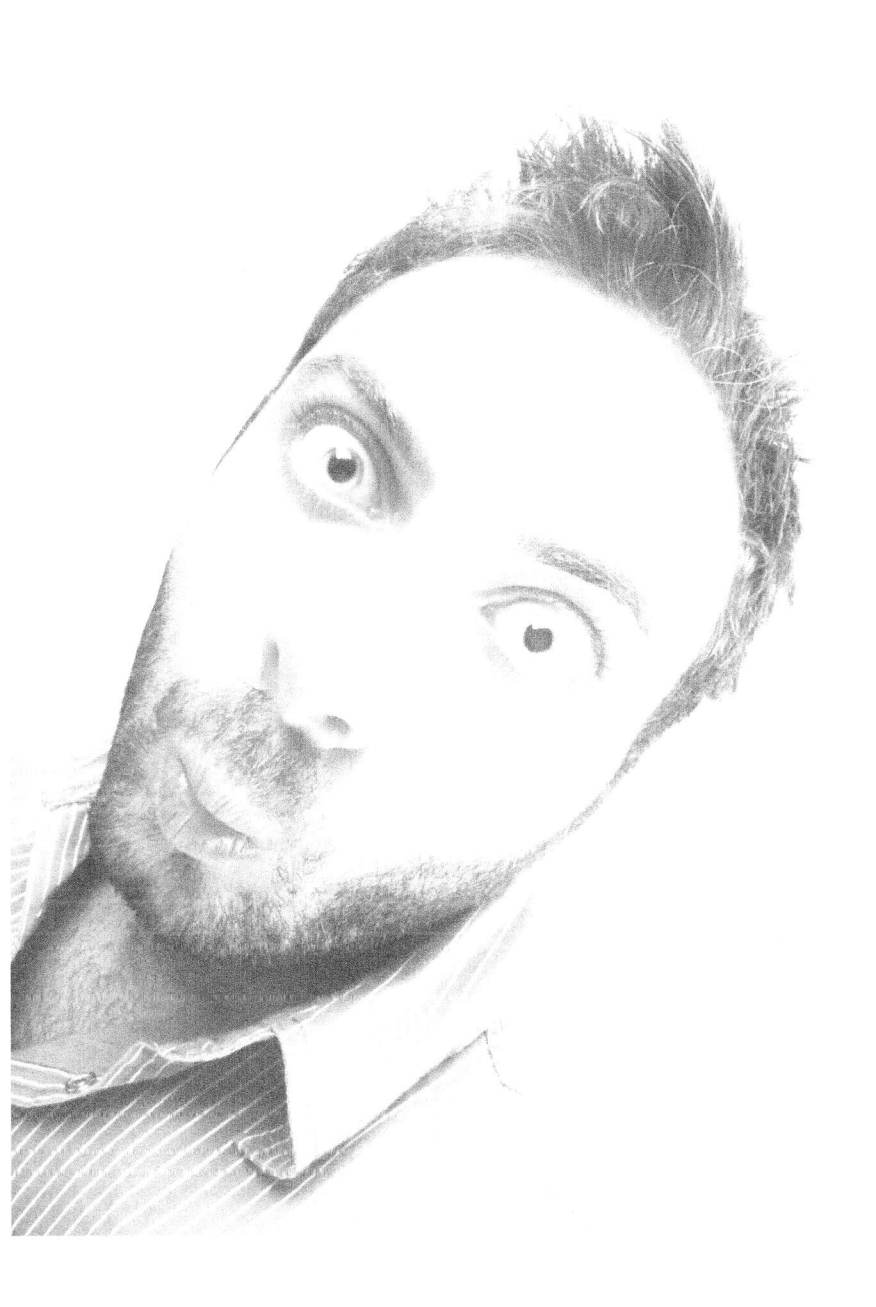

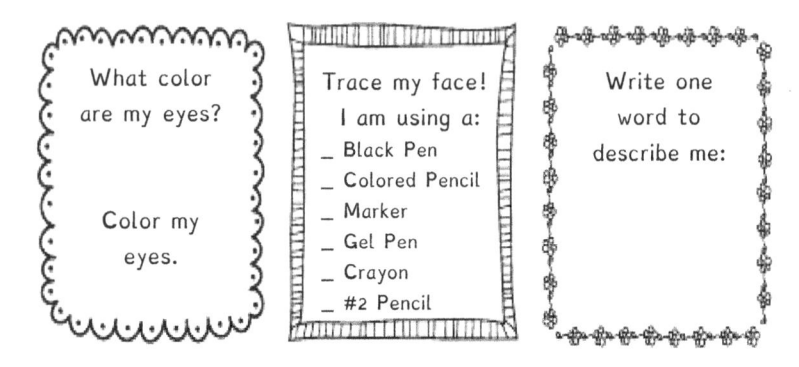

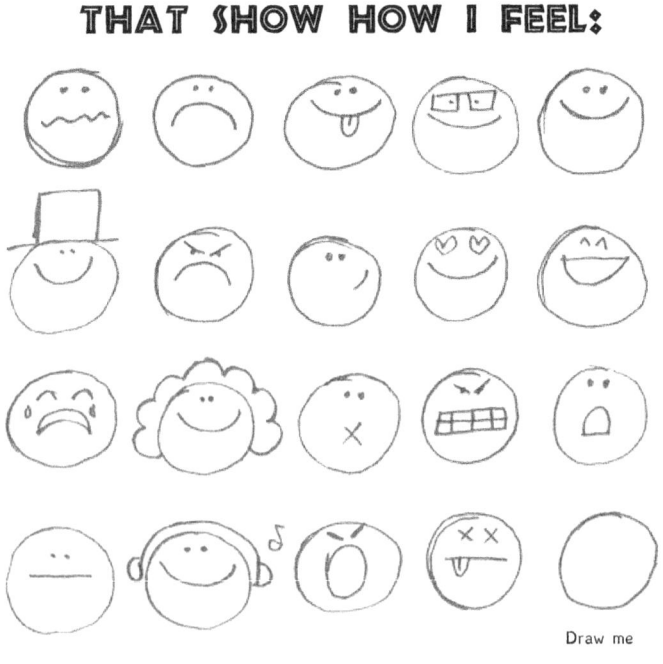

LOOK AT MY FACE!

What color are my eyes?

Color my eyes.

Trace my face!
I am using a:
- Black Pen
- Colored Pencil
- Marker
- Gel Pen
- Crayon
- #2 Pencil

Write one word to describe me:

COLOR THE FACES THAT SHOW HOW I FEEL:

Draw me

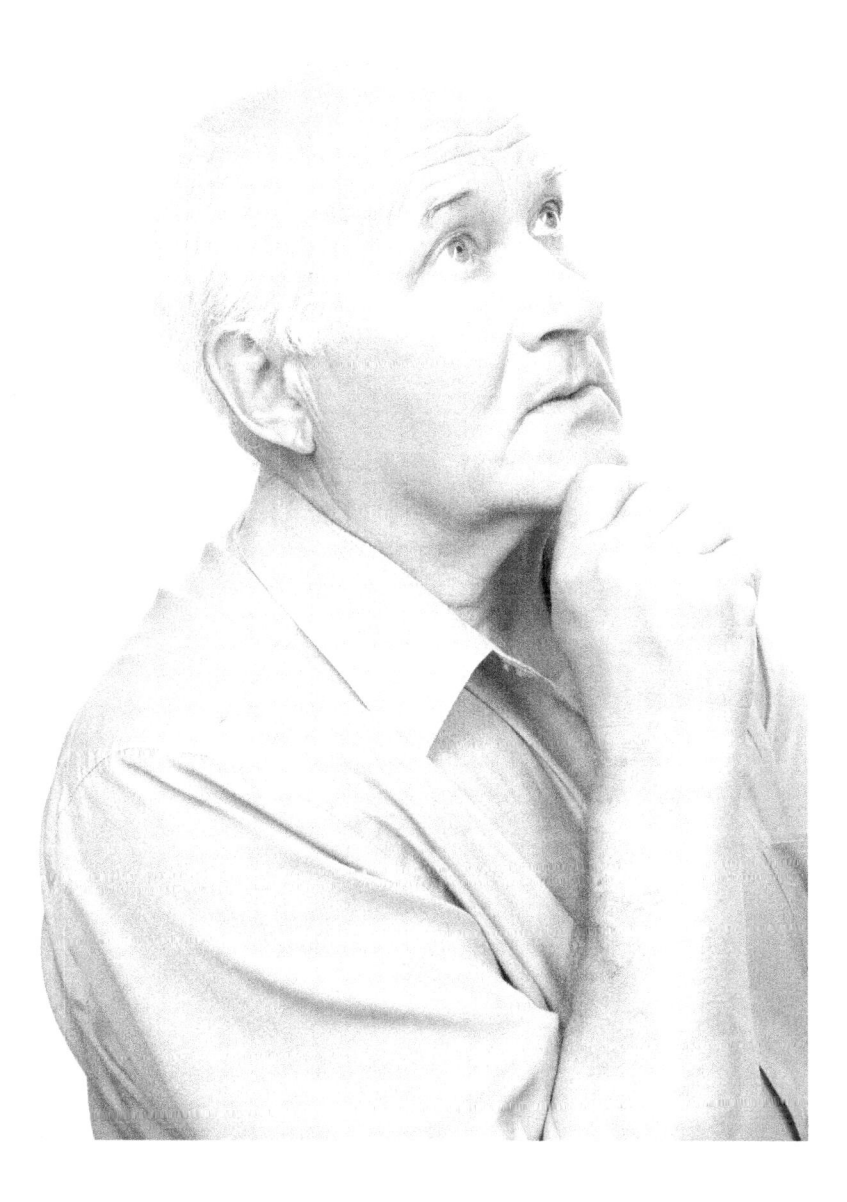

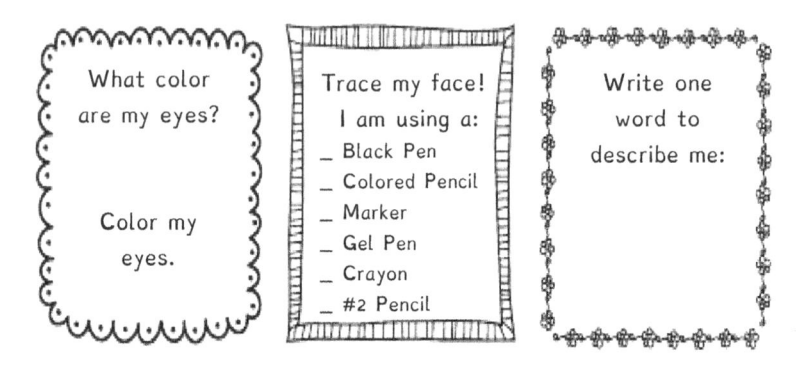

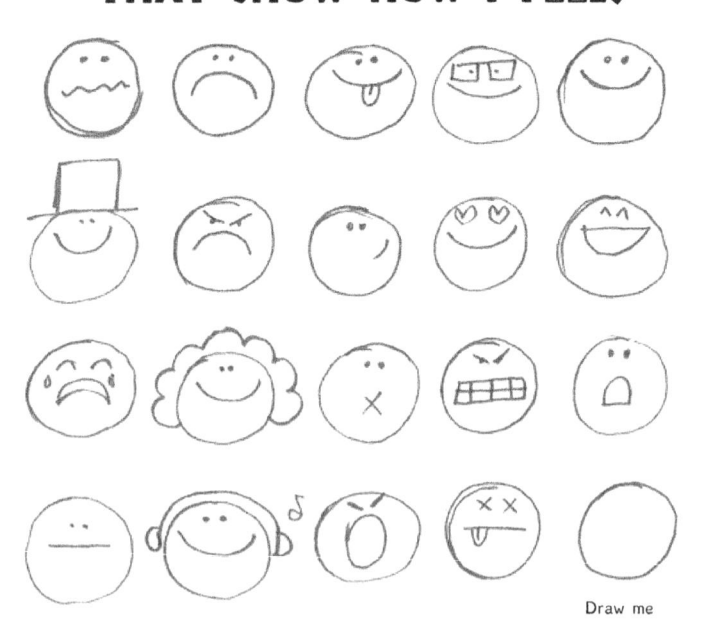

LOOK AT MY FACE!

What color are my eyes?

Color my eyes.

Trace my face!
I am using a:
_ Black Pen
_ Colored Pencil
_ Marker
_ Gel Pen
_ Crayon
_ #2 Pencil

Write one word to describe me:

COLOR THE FACES THAT SHOW HOW I FEEL:

Draw me

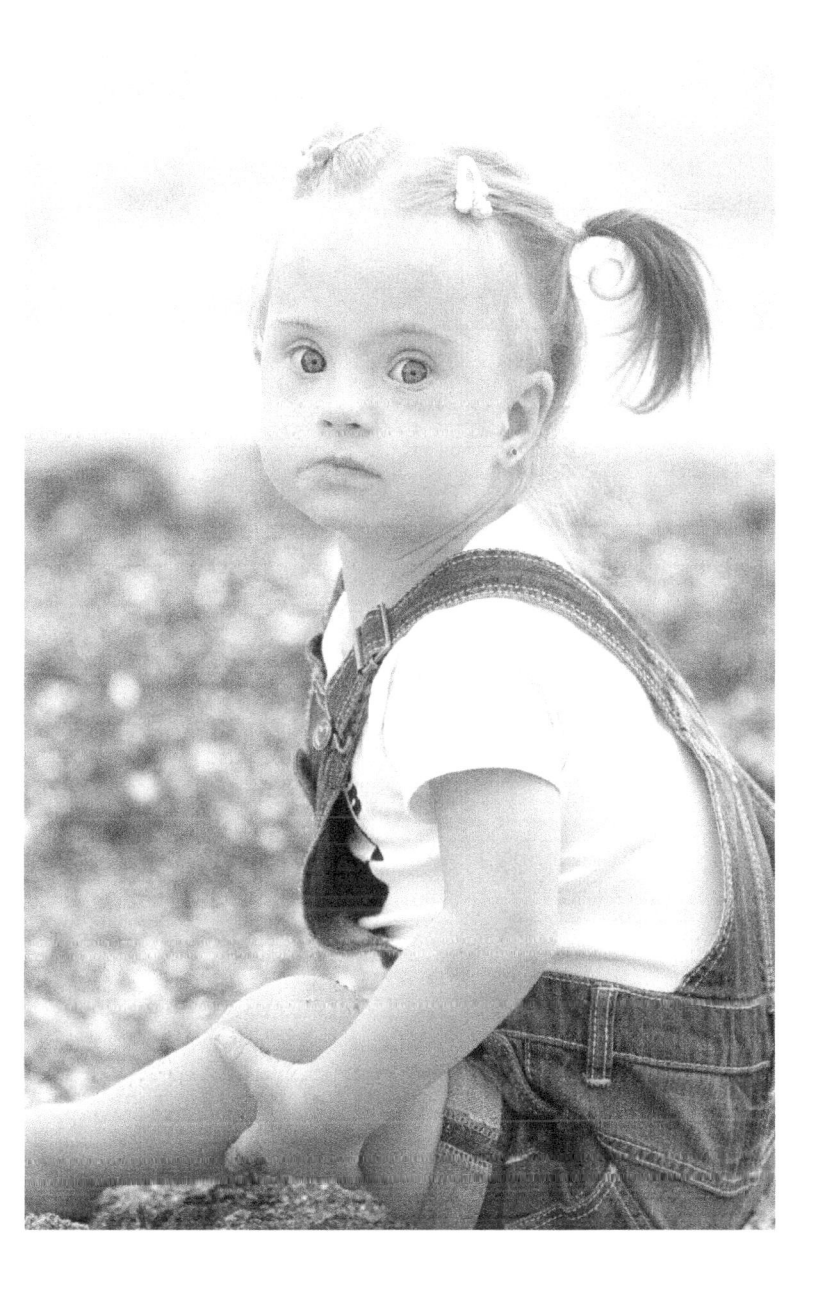

Today I am thinking about:

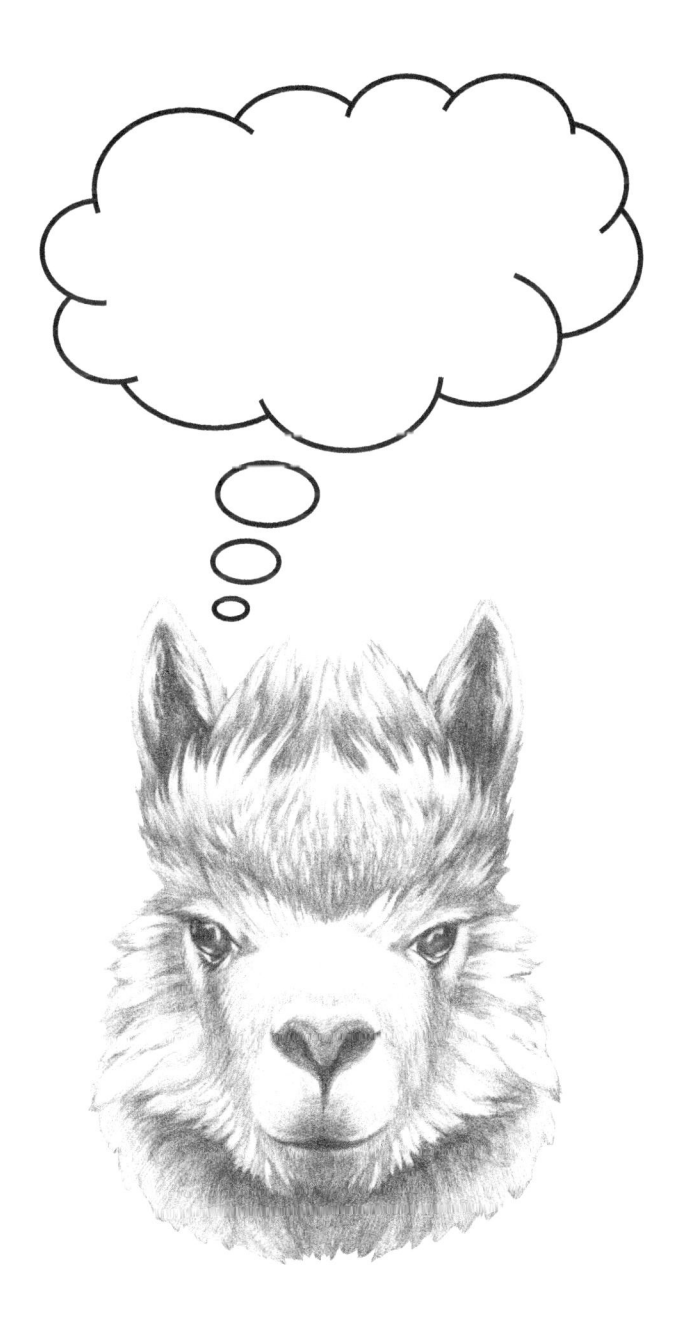

DRAW ANYTHING

LOGIC GAMES

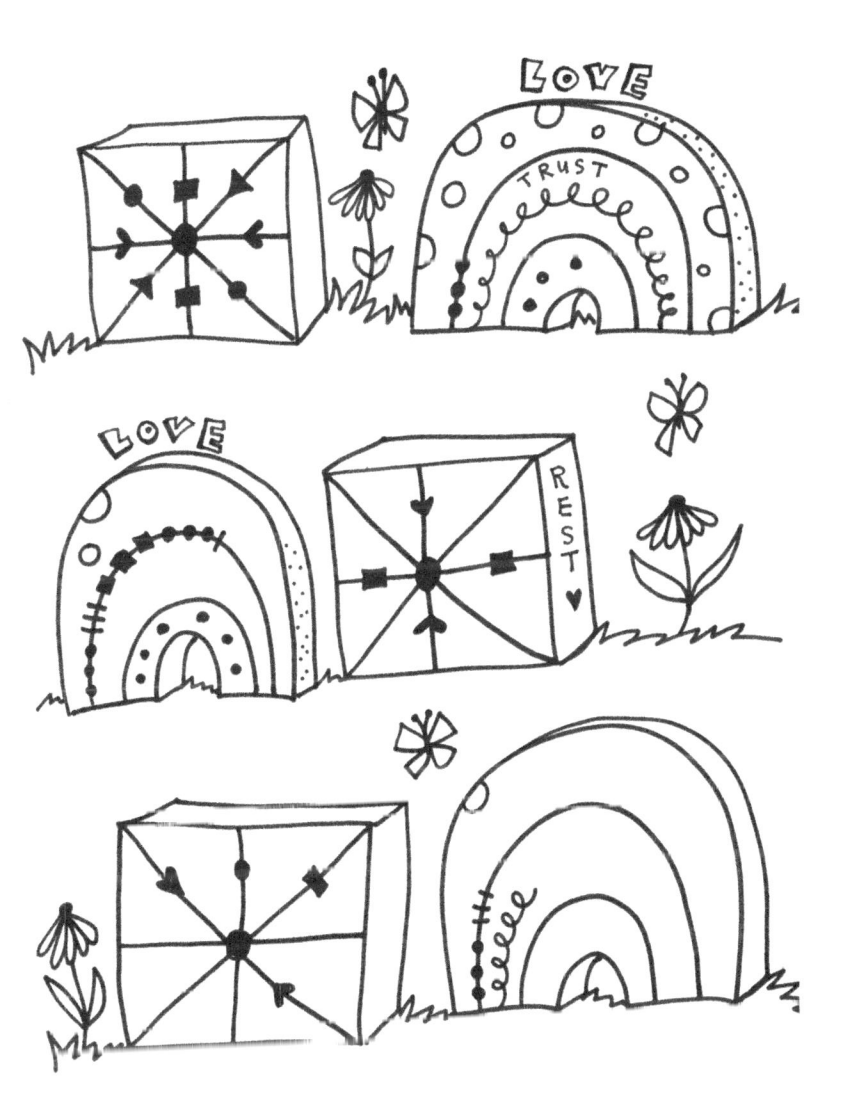

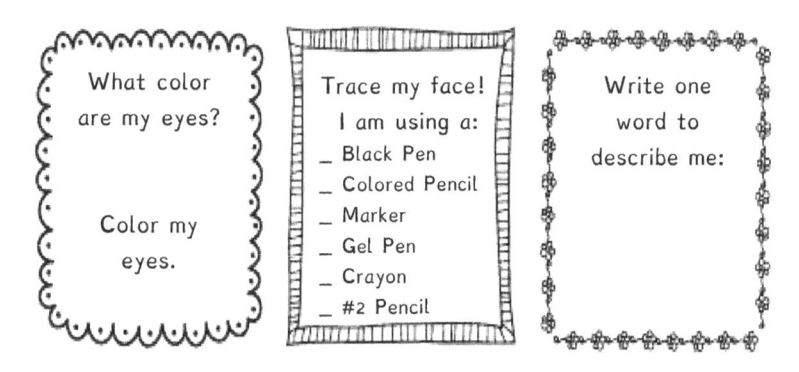

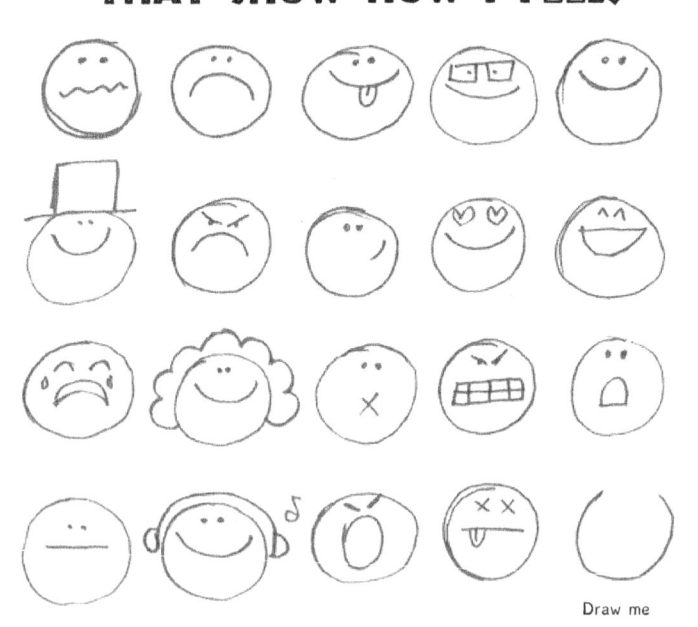

LOOK AT MY FACE!

What color are my eyes?

Color my eyes.

Trace my face!
I am using a:
_ Black Pen
_ Colored Pencil
_ Marker
_ Gel Pen
_ Crayon
_ #2 Pencil

Write one word to describe me:

COLOR THE FACES THAT SHOW HOW I FEEL:

Draw me

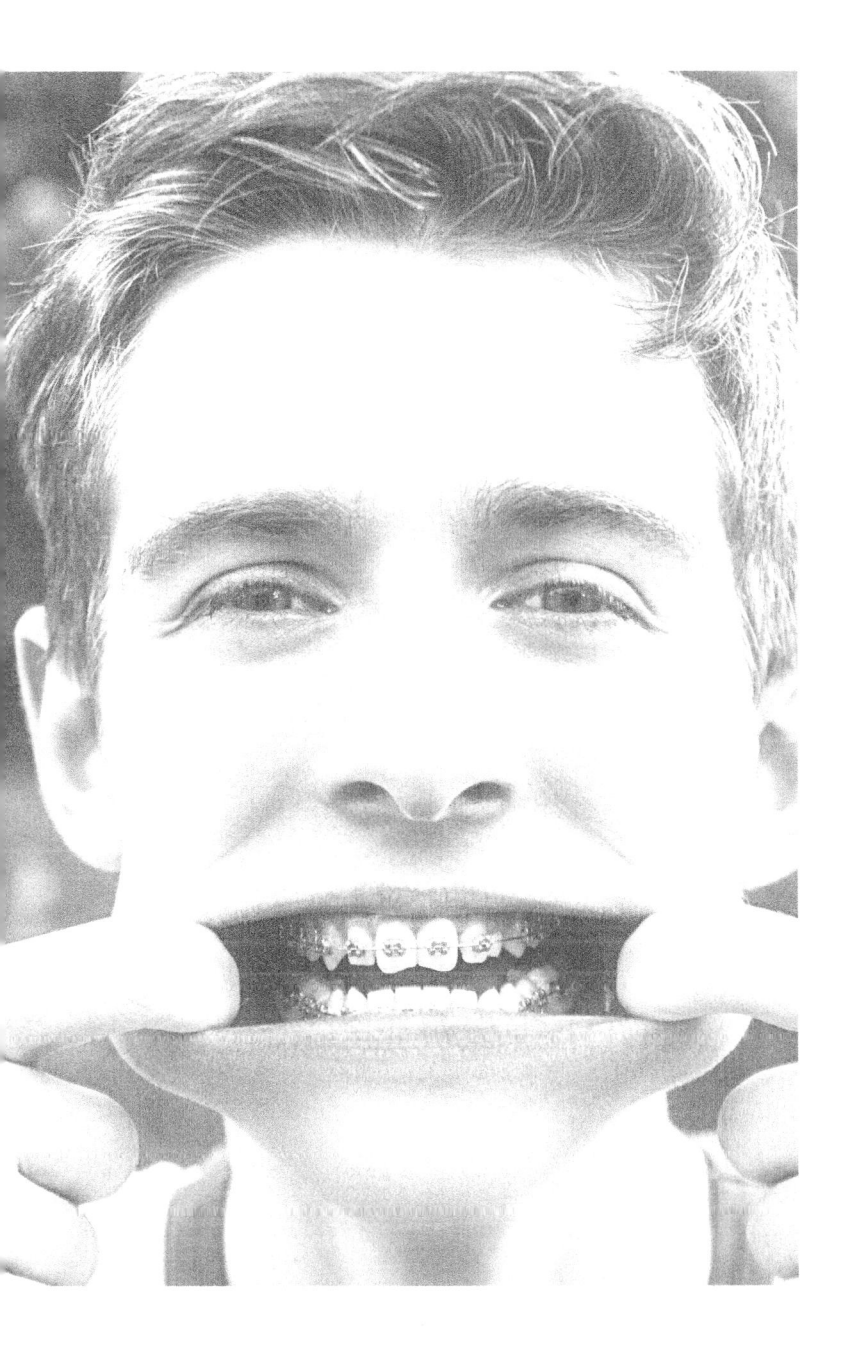

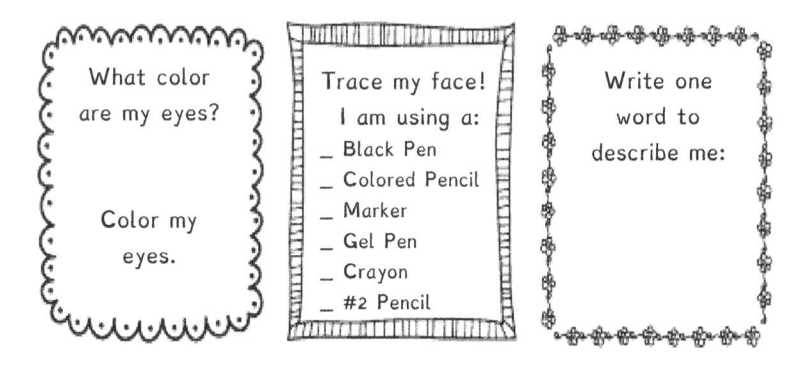

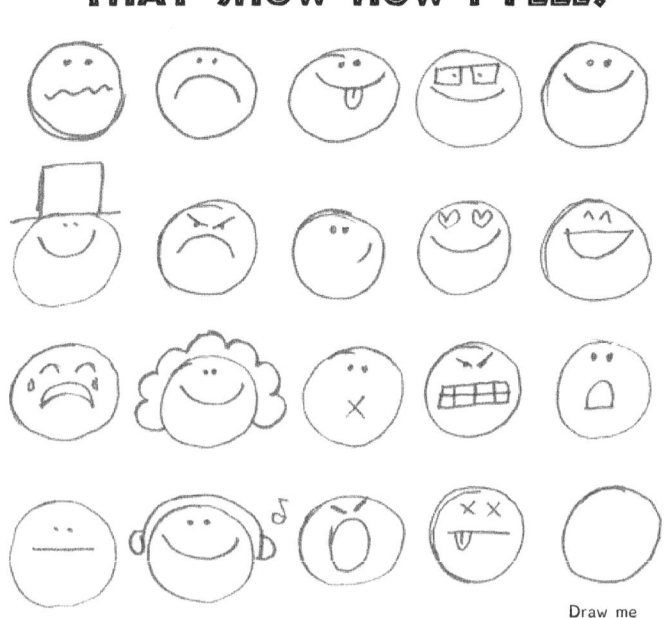

LOOK AT MY FACE!

What color are my eyes?

Color my eyes.

Trace my face!
I am using a:
- Black Pen
- Colored Pencil
- Marker
- Gel Pen
- Crayon
- #2 Pencil

Write one word to describe me:

COLOR THE FACES THAT SHOW HOW I FEEL:

Draw me

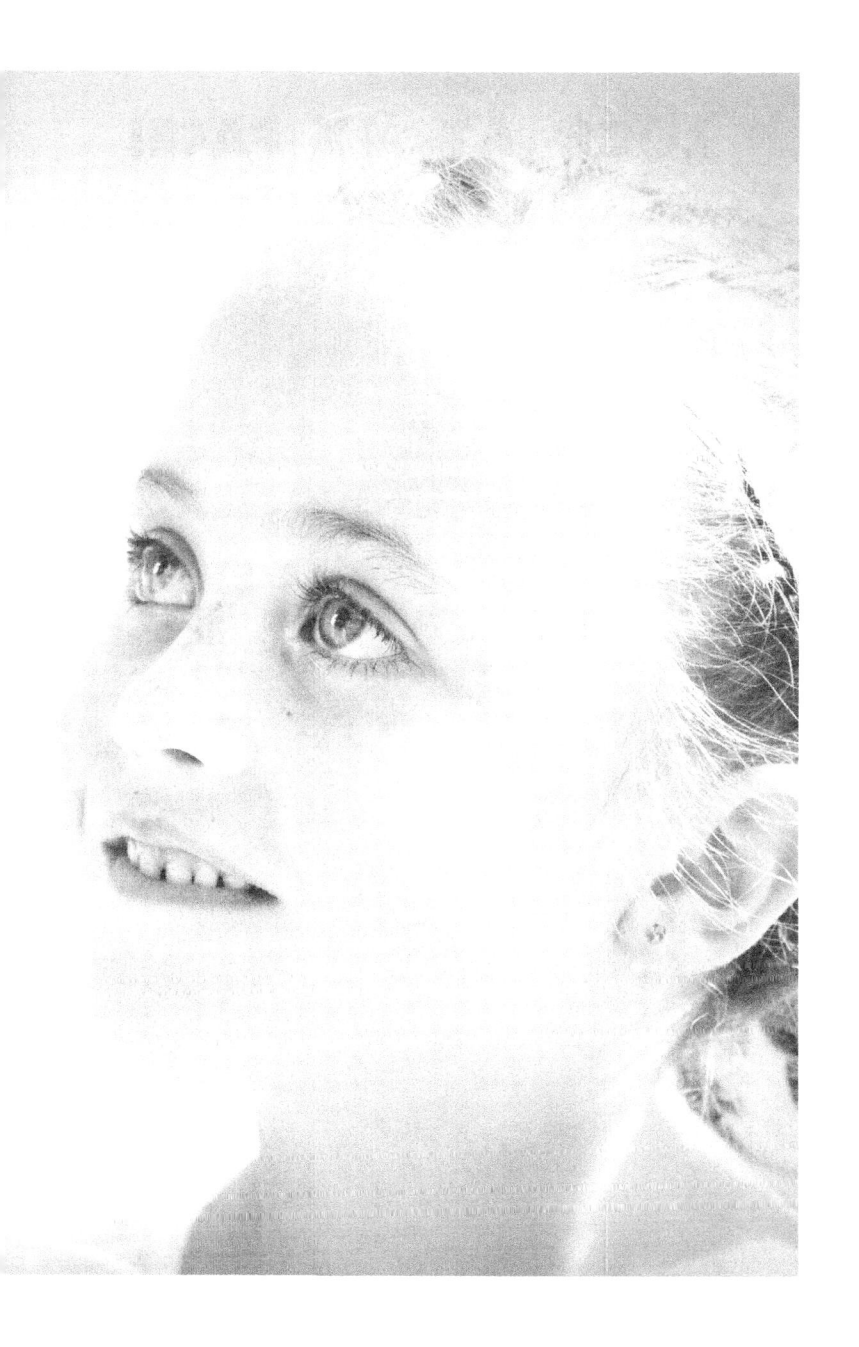

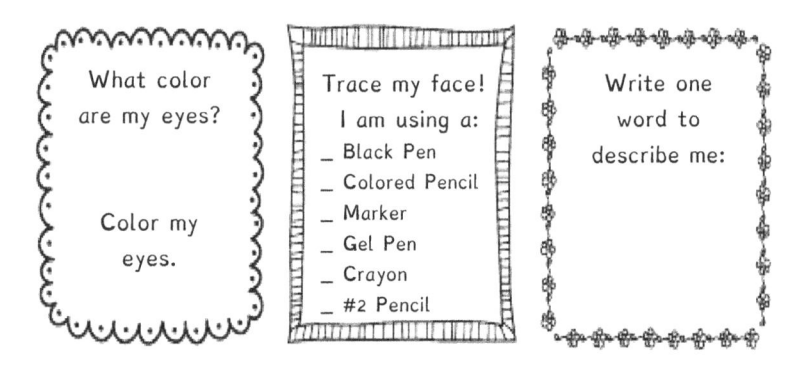

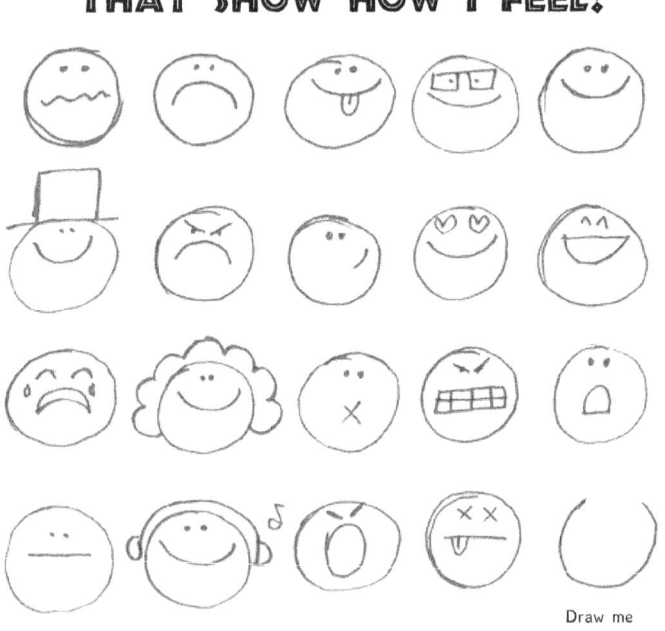

LOOK AT MY FACE!

What color are my eyes?

Color my eyes.

Trace my face!
I am using a:
_ Black Pen
_ Colored Pencil
_ Marker
_ Gel Pen
_ Crayon
_ #2 Pencil

Write one word to describe me:

COLOR THE FACES THAT SHOW HOW I FEEL:

Draw me

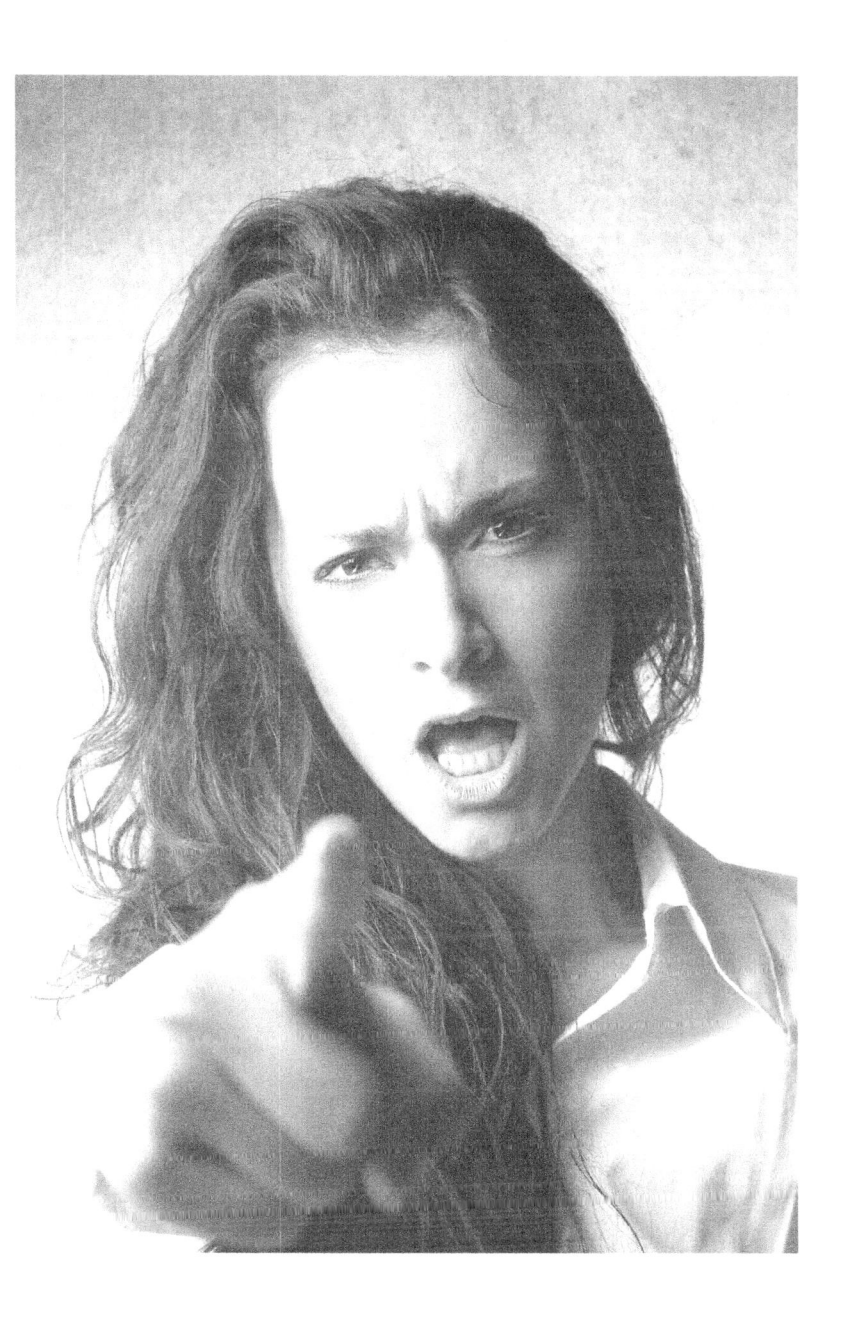

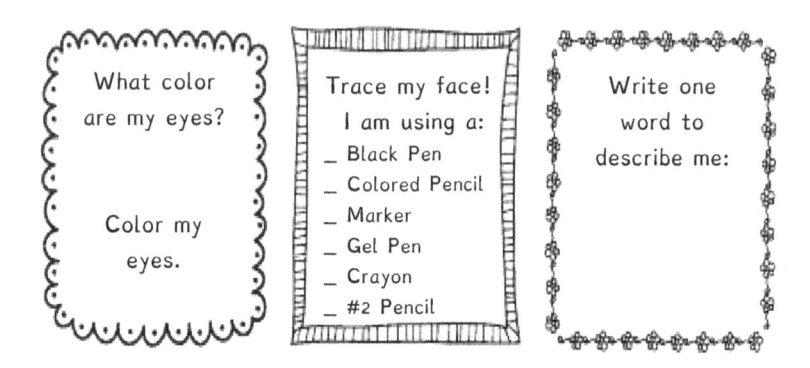

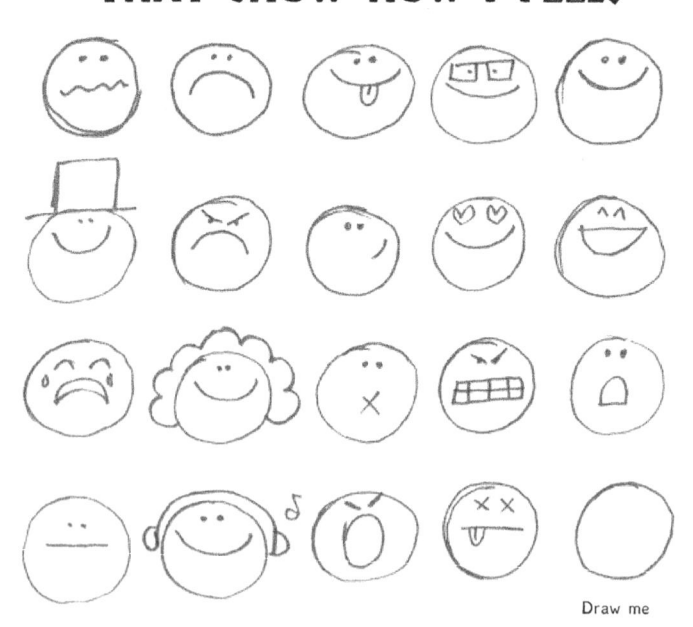

LOOK AT MY FACE!

What color are my eyes?

Color my eyes.

Trace my face!
I am using a:
- Black Pen
- Colored Pencil
- Marker
- Gel Pen
- Crayon
- #2 Pencil

Write one word to describe me:

COLOR THE FACES THAT SHOW HOW I FEEL:

Draw me

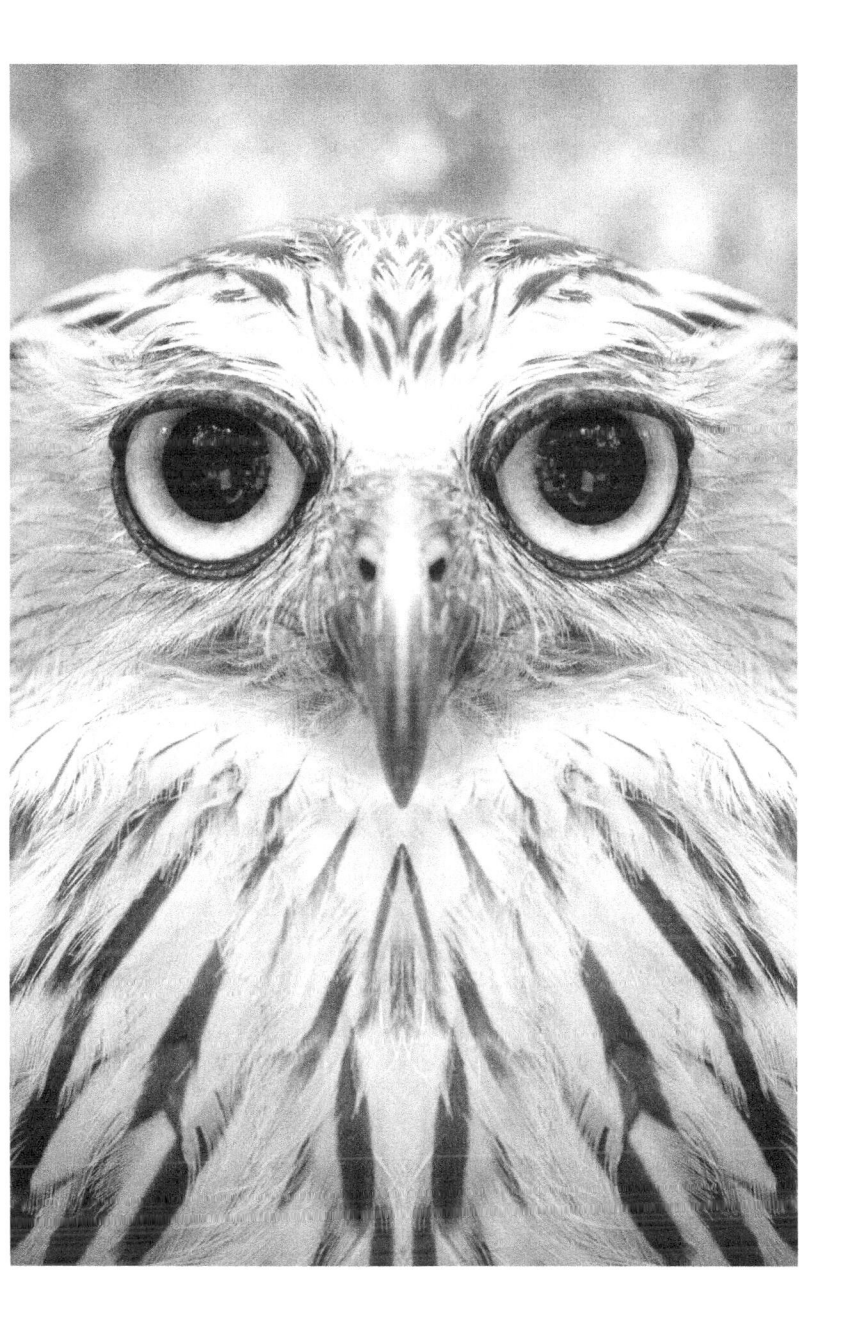

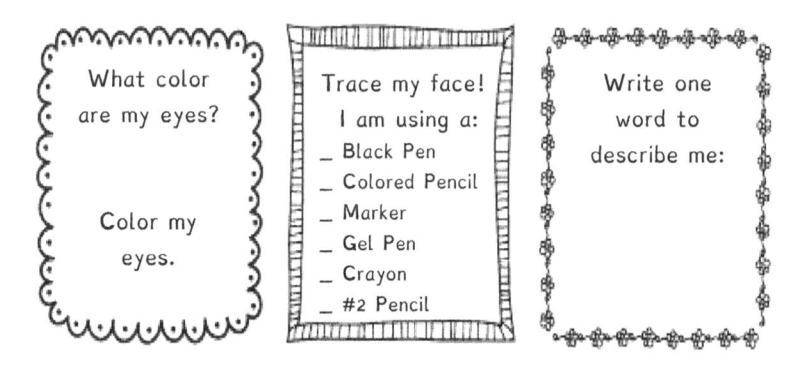

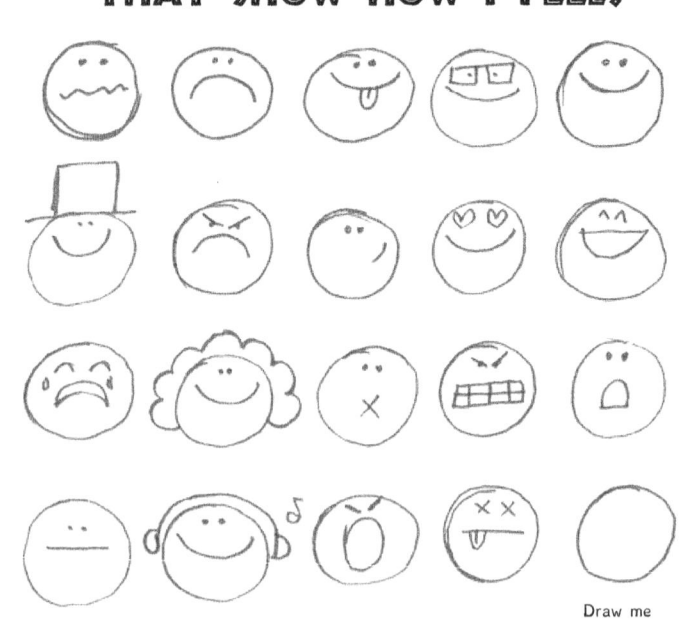

LOOK AT MY FACE!

What color are my eyes?

Color my eyes.

Trace my face! I am using a:
_ Black Pen
_ Colored Pencil
_ Marker
_ Gel Pen
_ Crayon
_ #2 Pencil

Write one word to describe me:

COLOR THE FACES THAT SHOW HOW I FEEL:

Draw me

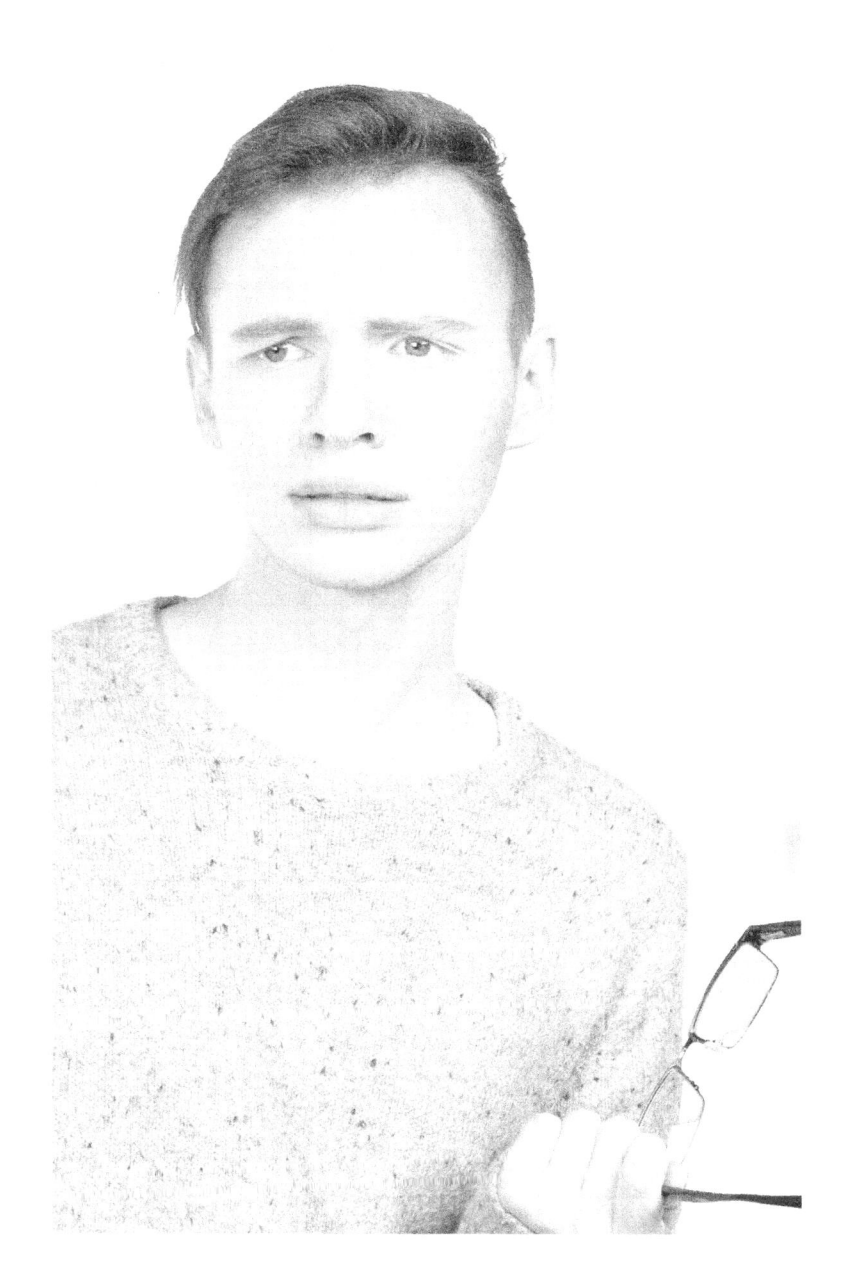

Today I am thinking about:

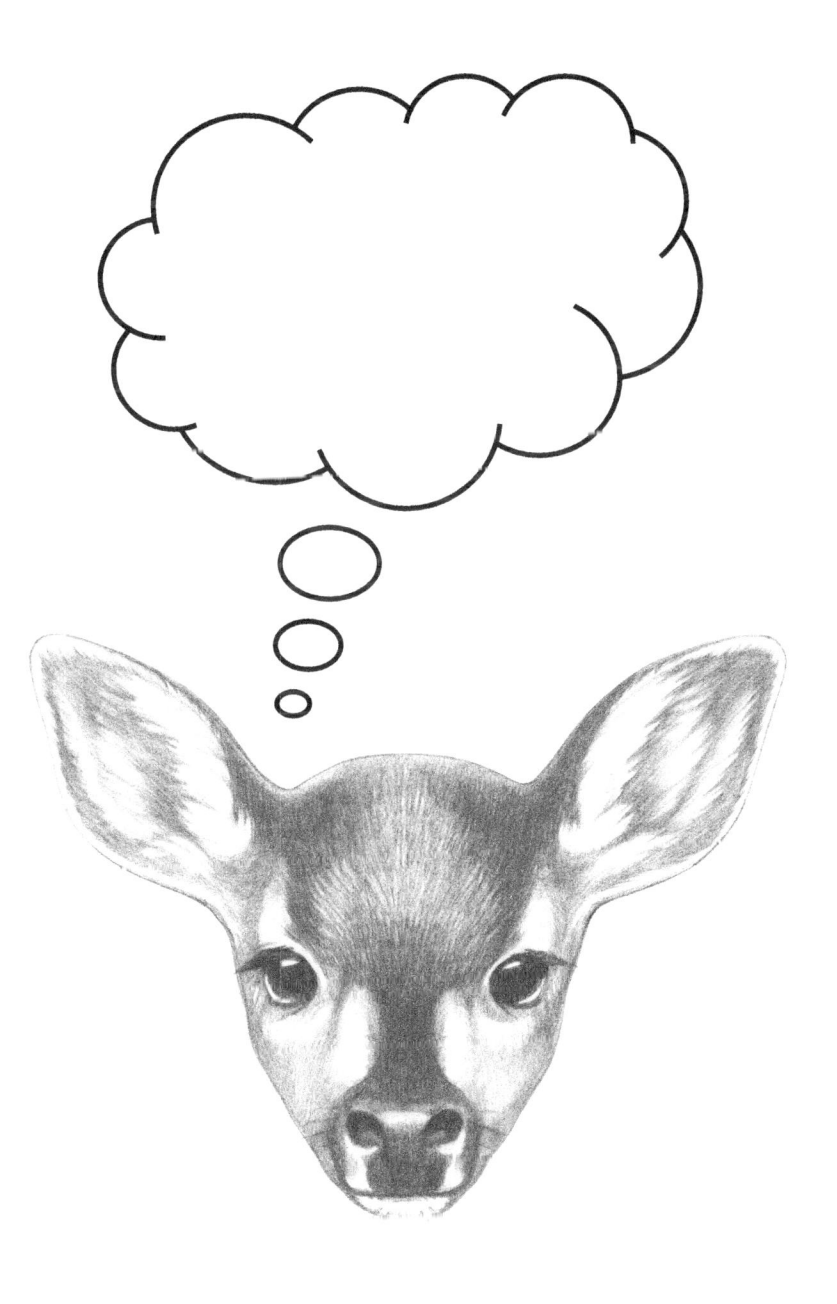

DRAW ANYTHING

LOGIC GAMES

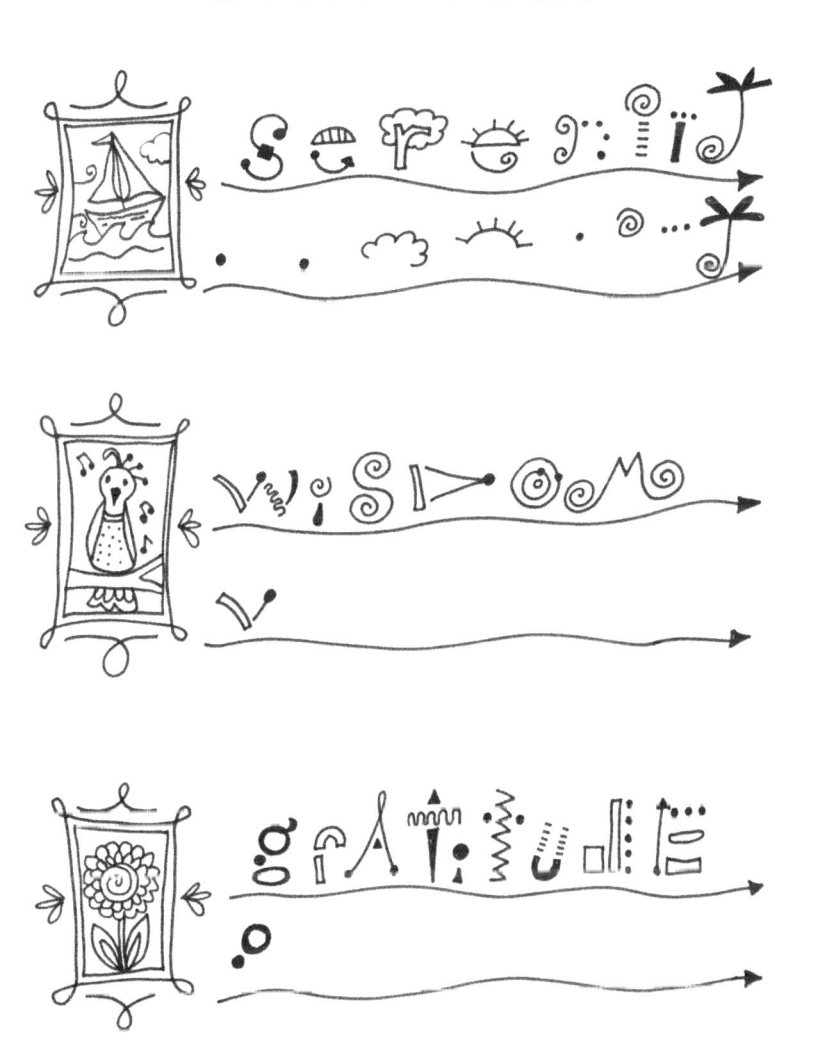

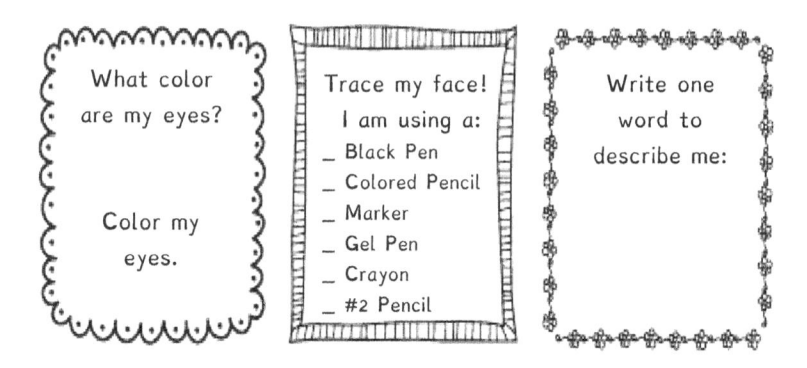

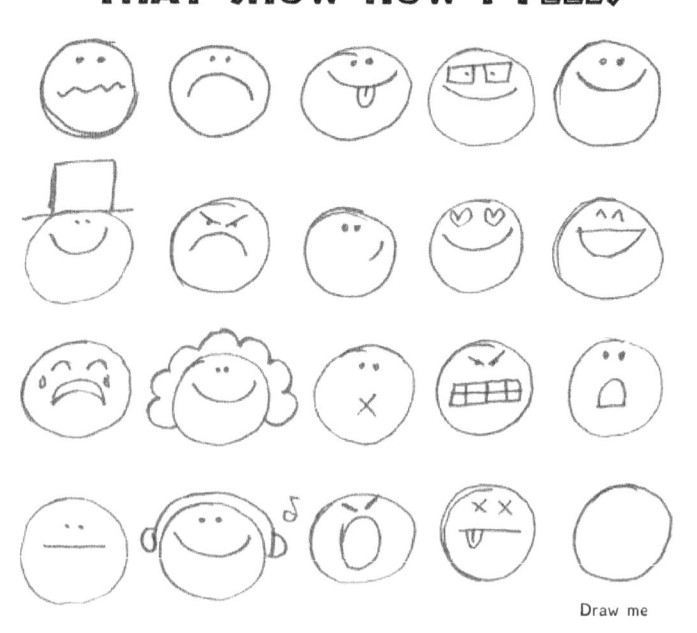

LOOK AT MY FACE!

What color are my eyes?

Color my eyes.

Trace my face!
I am using a:
_ Black Pen
_ Colored Pencil
_ Marker
_ Gel Pen
_ Crayon
_ #2 Pencil

Write one word to describe me:

COLOR THE FACES THAT SHOW HOW I FEEL:

Draw me

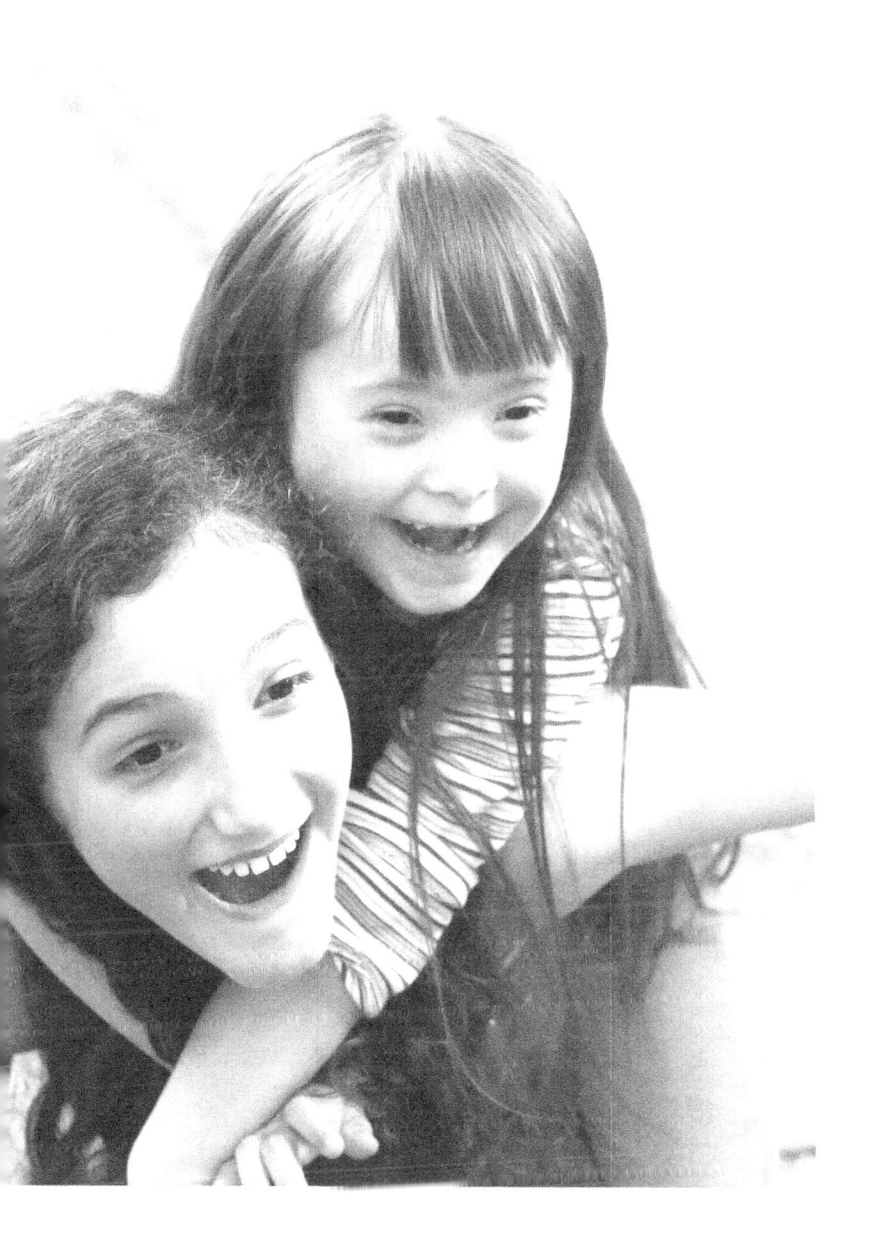

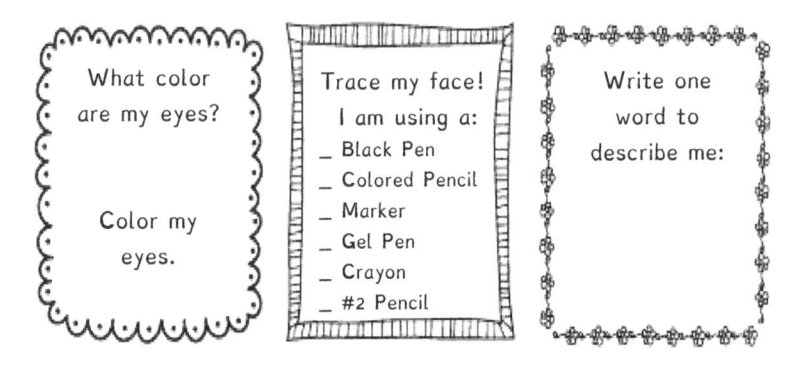

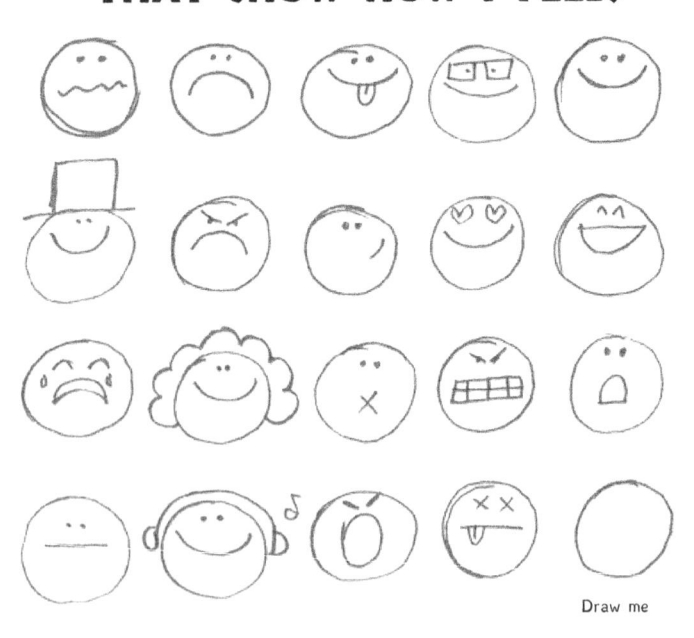

LOOK AT MY FACE!

| What color are my eyes? Color my eyes. | Trace my face! I am using a: _ Black Pen _ Colored Pencil _ Marker _ Gel Pen _ Crayon _ #2 Pencil | Write one word to describe me: |

COLOR THE FACES THAT SHOW HOW I FEEL:

Draw me

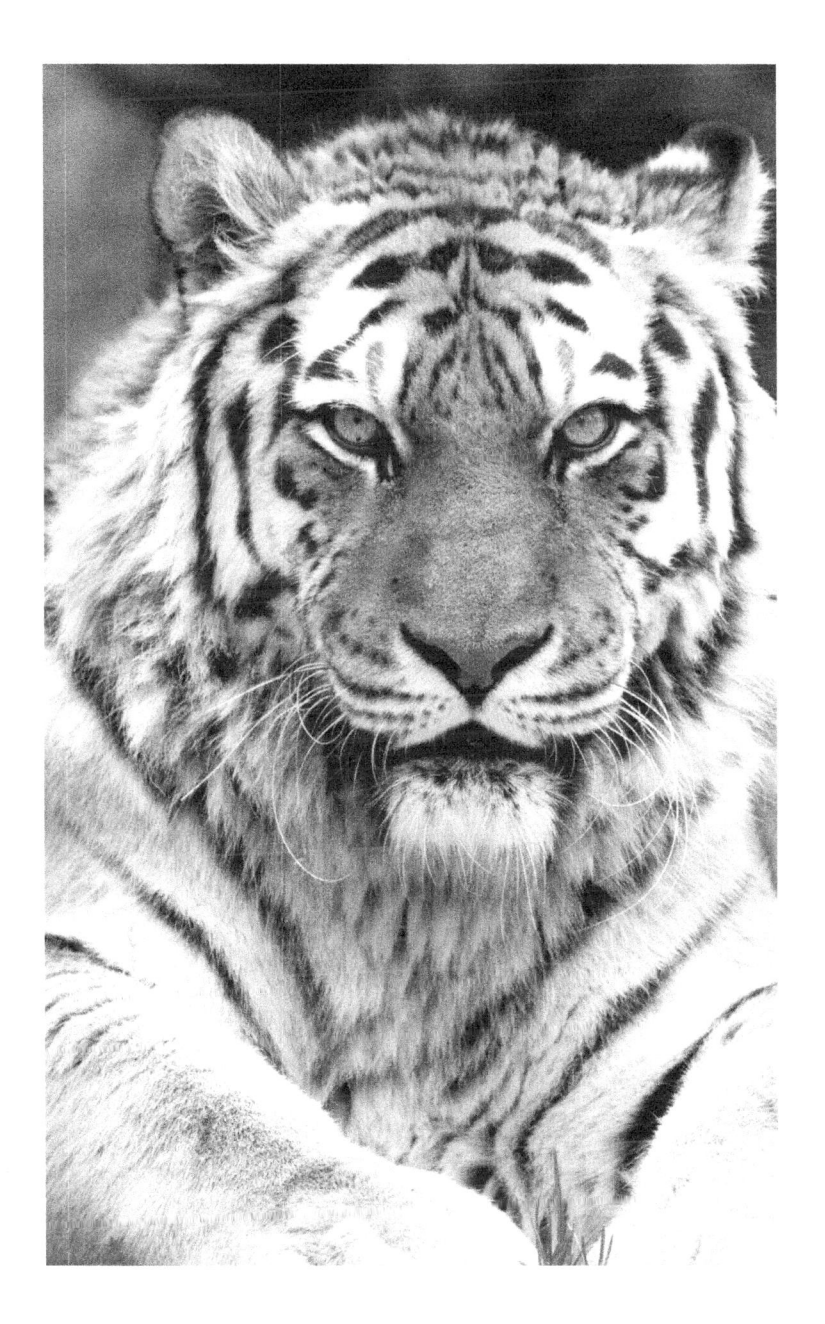

LOOK AT MY FACE!

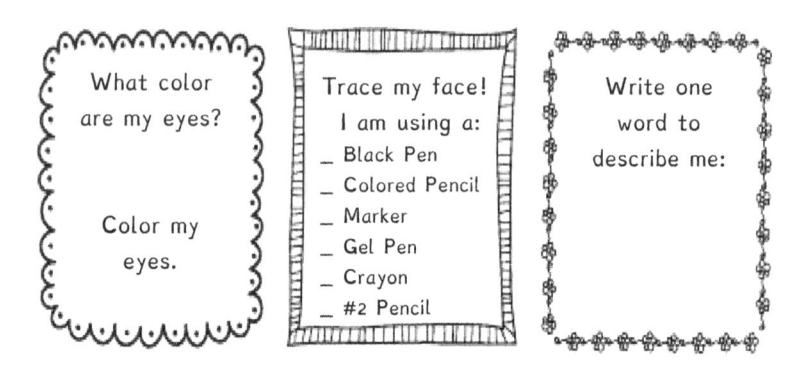

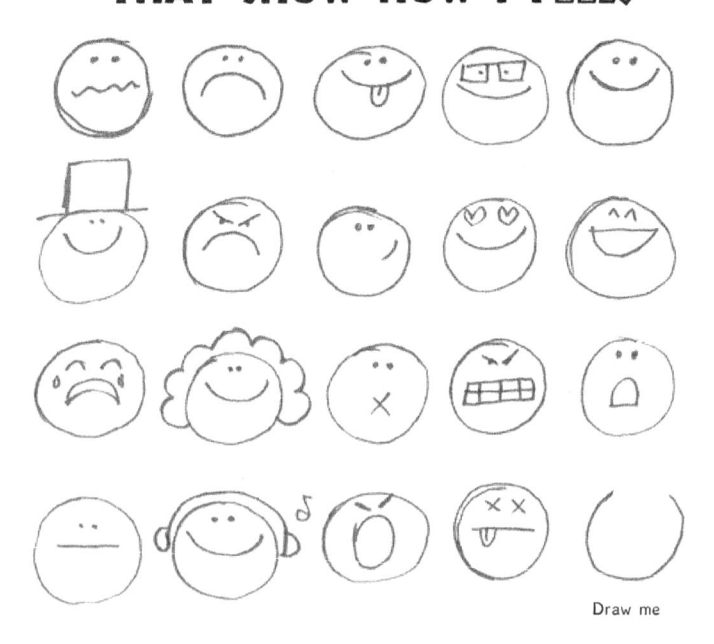

What color are my eyes?

Color my eyes.

Trace my face!
I am using a:
- _ Black Pen
- _ Colored Pencil
- _ Marker
- _ Gel Pen
- _ Crayon
- _ #2 Pencil

Write one word to describe me:

COLOR THE FACES THAT SHOW HOW I FEEL:

Draw me

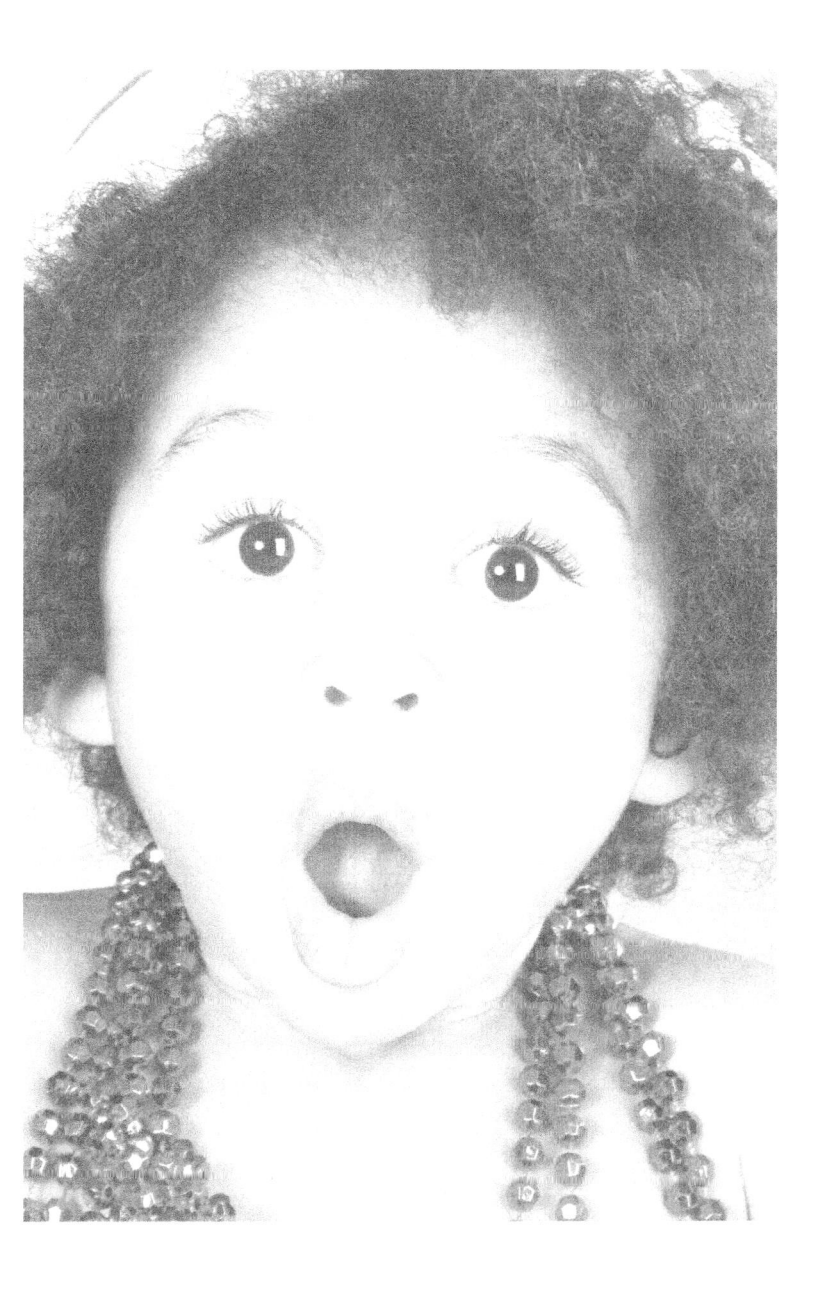

LOOK AT MY FACE!

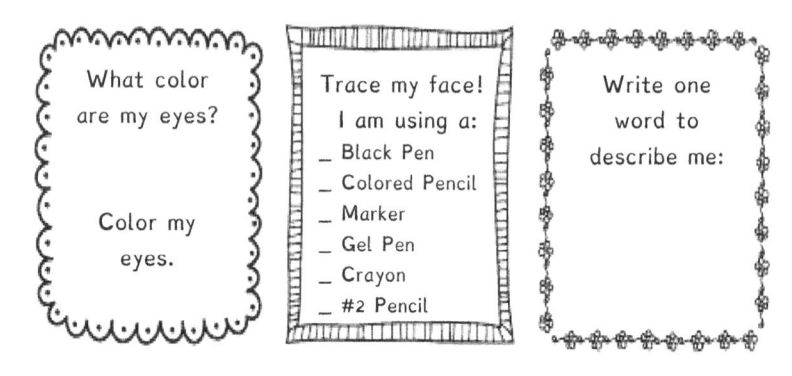

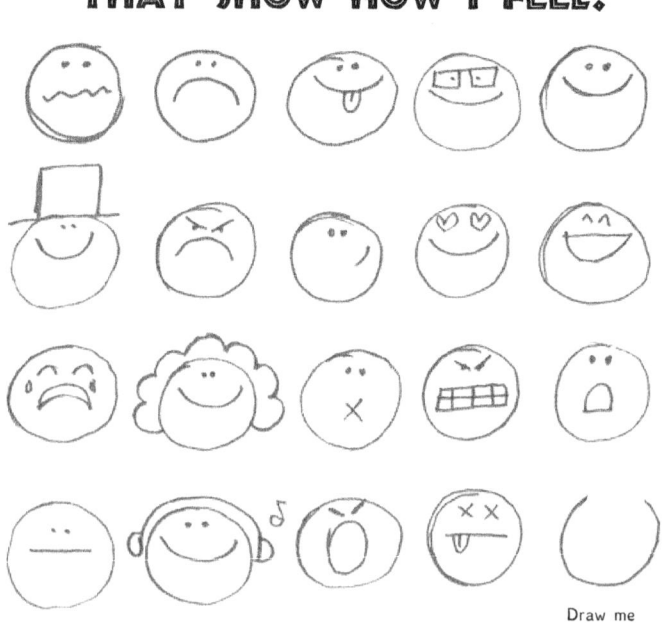

What color are my eyes?

Color my eyes.

Trace my face!
I am using a:
- Black Pen
- Colored Pencil
- Marker
- Gel Pen
- Crayon
- #2 Pencil

Write one word to describe me:

COLOR THE FACES THAT SHOW HOW I FEEL:

Draw me

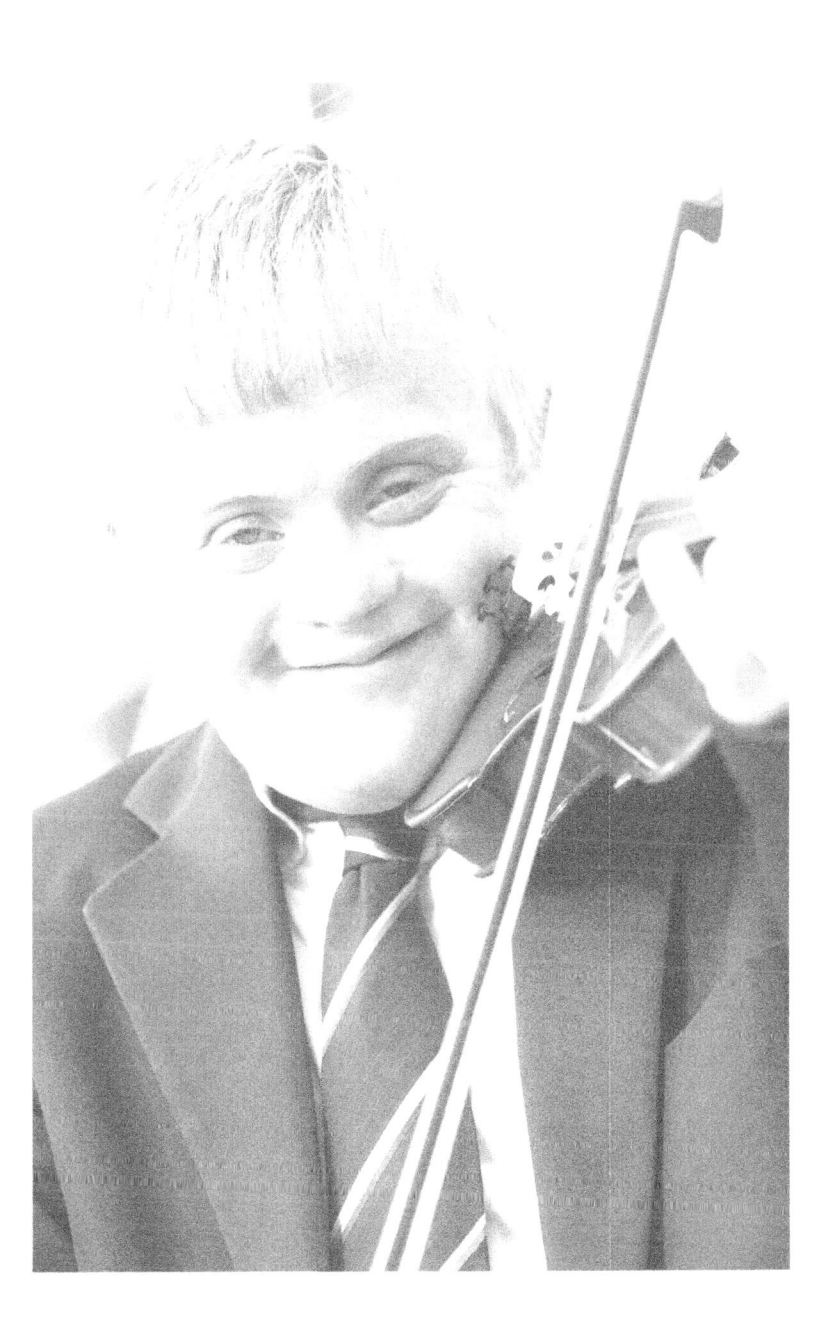

LOOK AT MY FACE!

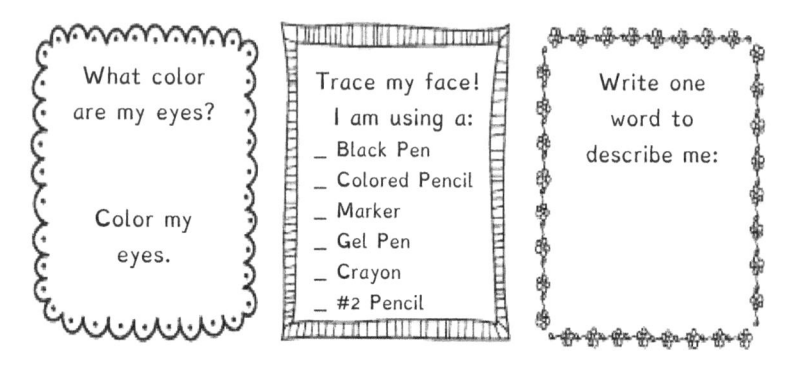

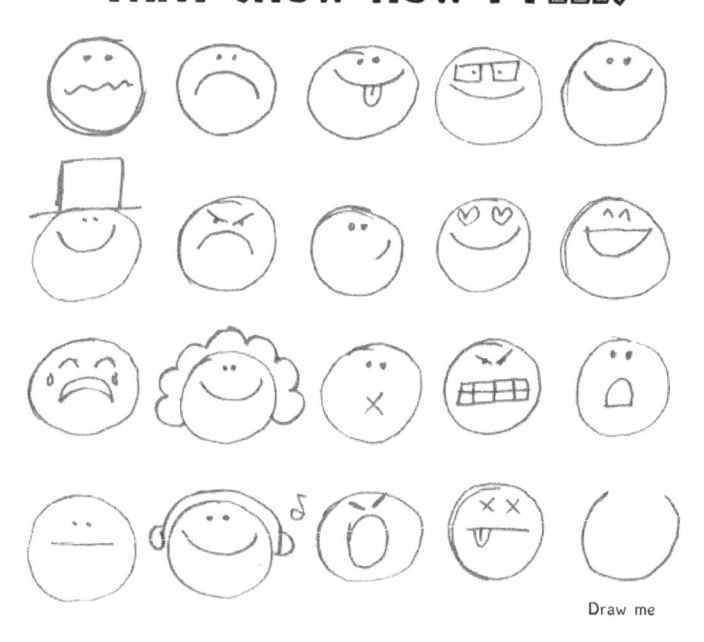

What color are my eyes?

Color my eyes.

Trace my face!
I am using a:
- Black Pen
- Colored Pencil
- Marker
- Gel Pen
- Crayon
- #2 Pencil

Write one word to describe me:

COLOR THE FACES THAT SHOW HOW I FEEL:

Draw me

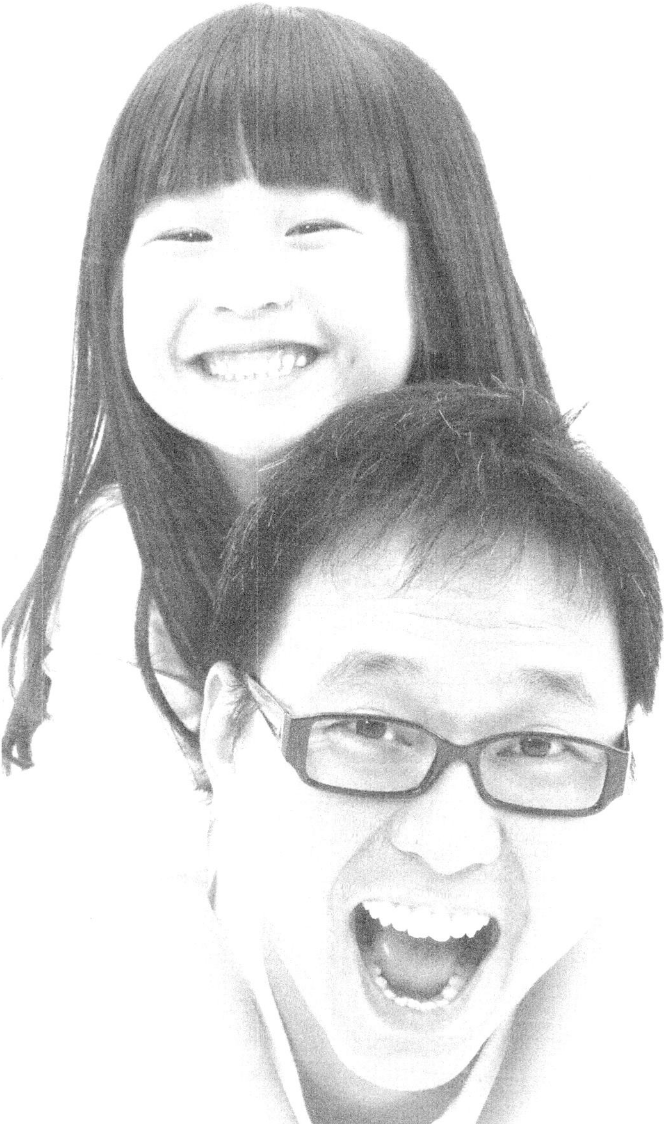

Today I am thinking about:

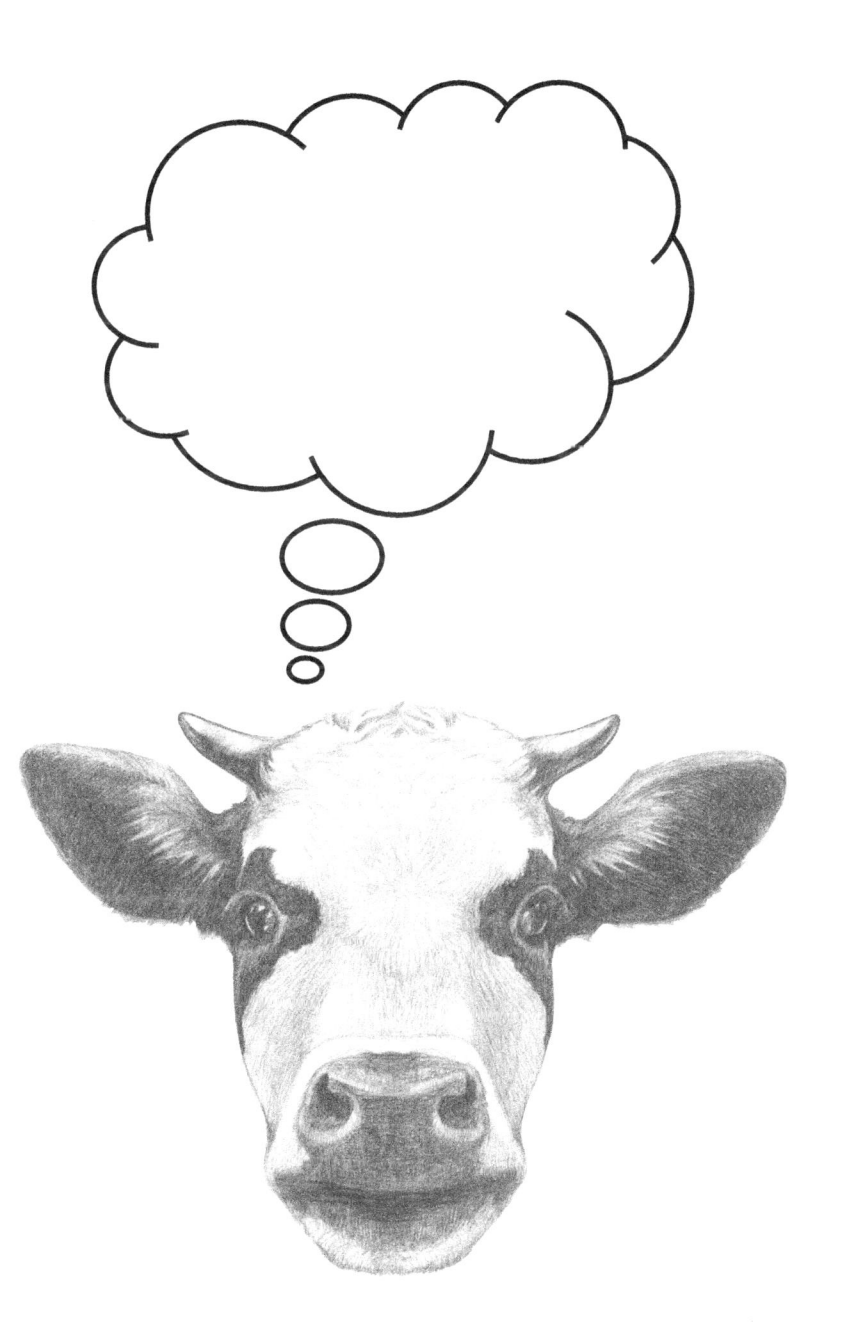

DRAW ANYTHING

LOGIC GAMES

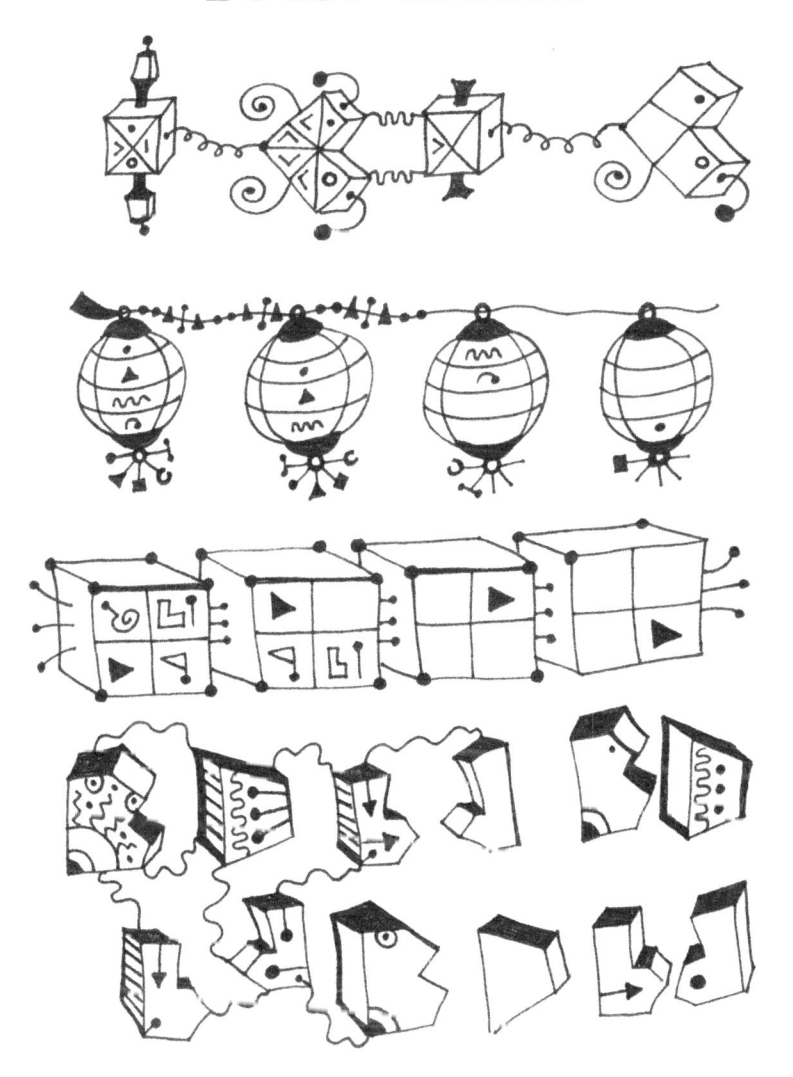

LOOK AT MY FACE!

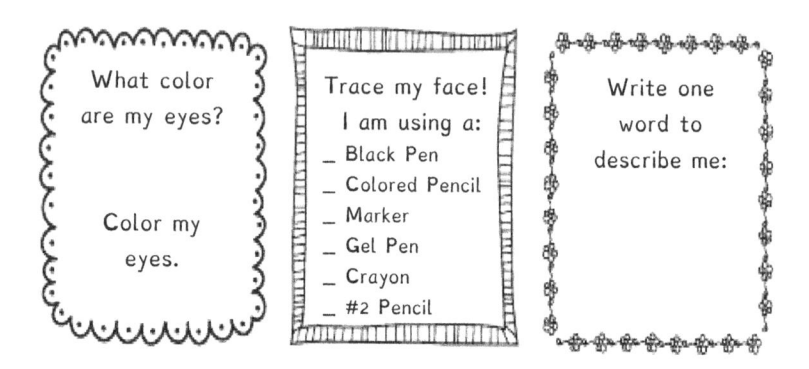

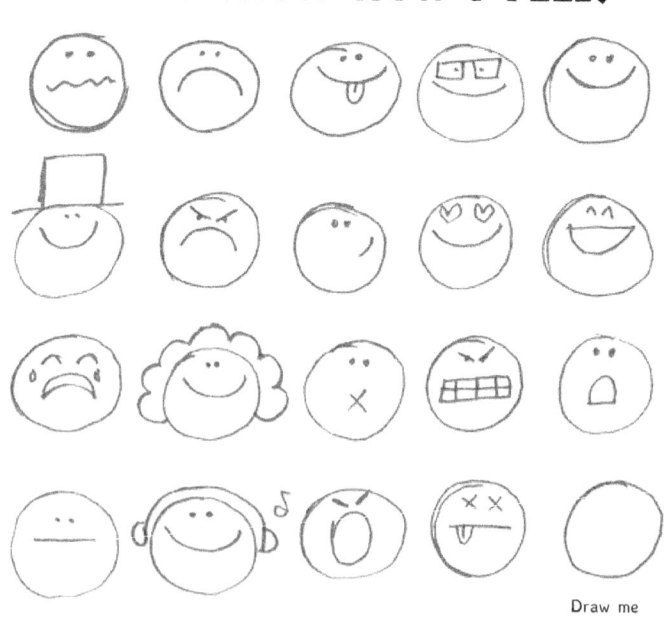

What color are my eyes?

Color my eyes.

Trace my face!
I am using a:
_ Black Pen
_ Colored Pencil
_ Marker
_ Gel Pen
_ Crayon
_ #2 Pencil

Write one word to describe me:

COLOR THE FACES THAT SHOW HOW I FEEL:

Draw me

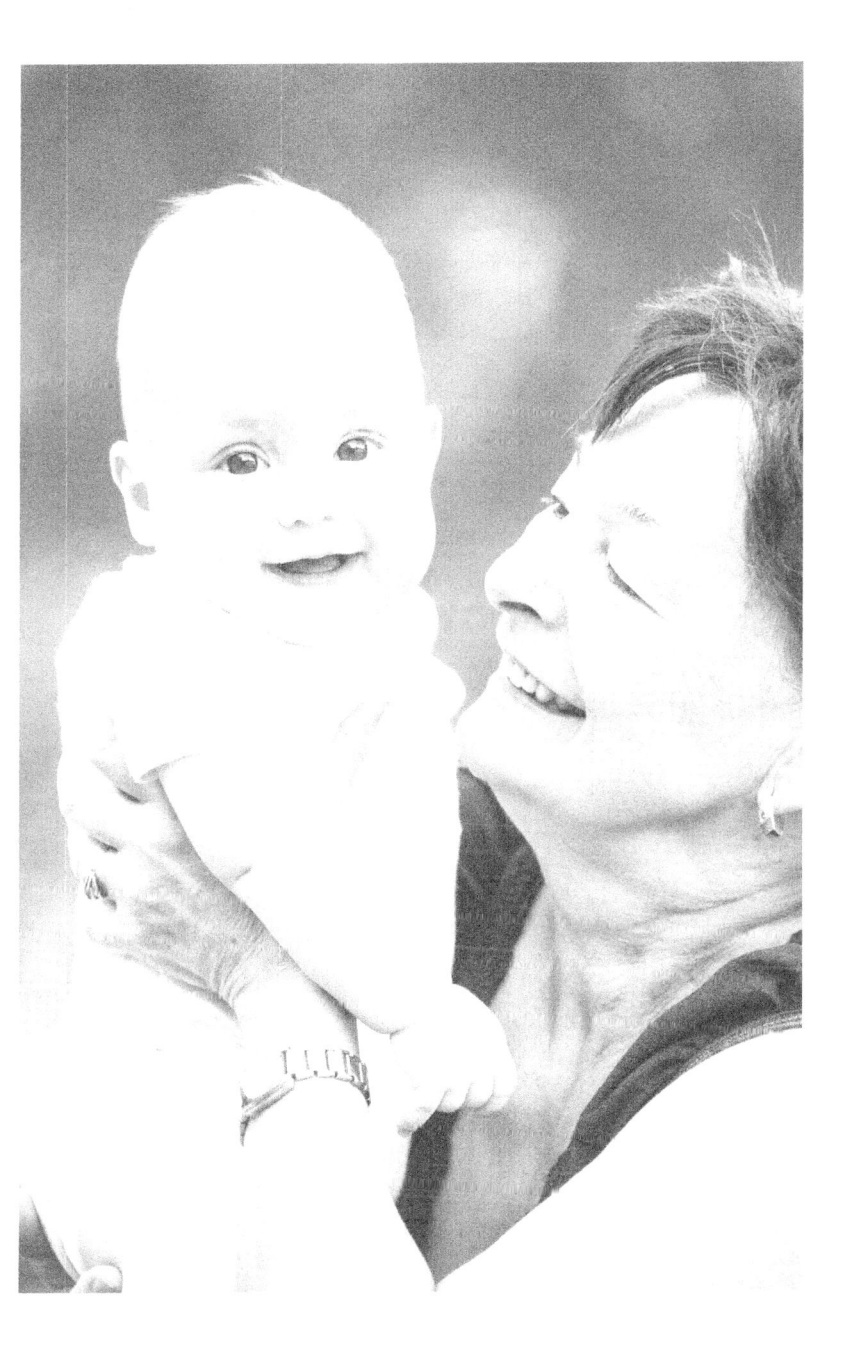

LOOK AT MY FACE!

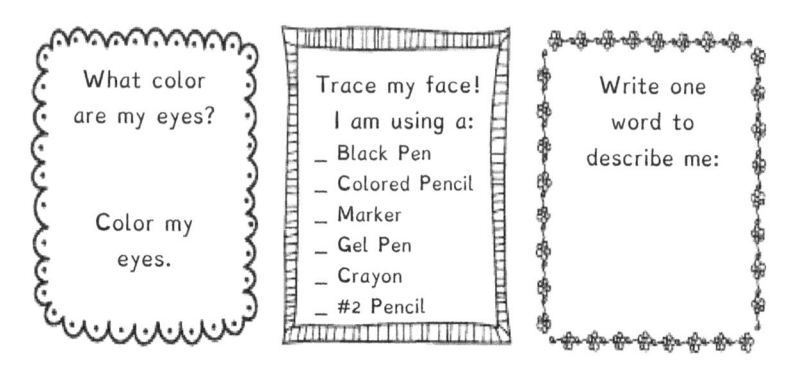

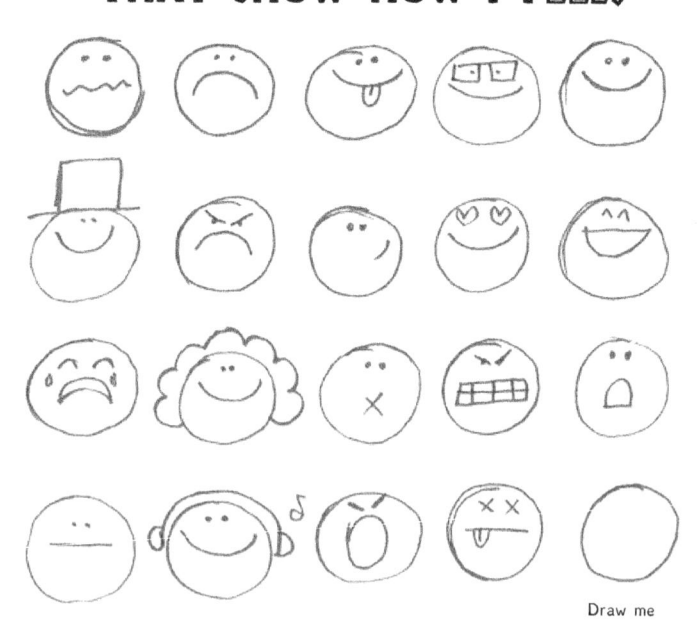

What color are my eyes?	Trace my face!	Write one word to describe me:
Color my eyes.	I am using a: _ Black Pen _ Colored Pencil _ Marker _ Gel Pen _ Crayon _ #2 Pencil	

COLOR THE FACES THAT SHOW HOW I FEEL:

Draw me

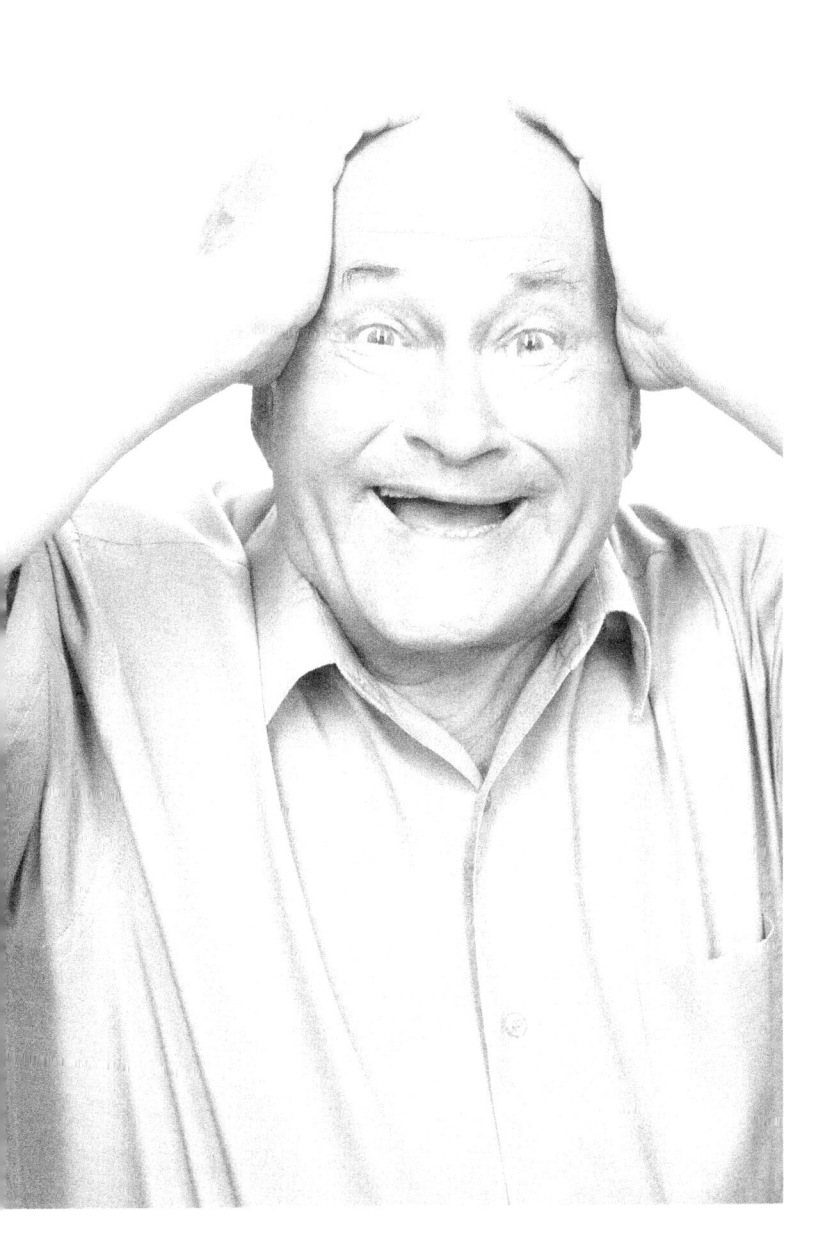

LOOK AT MY FACE!

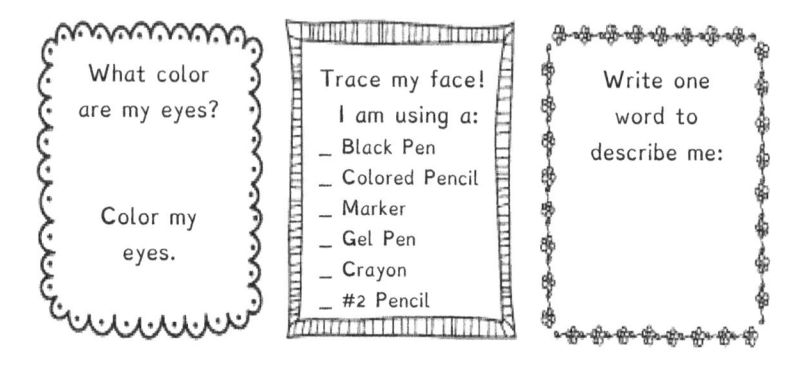

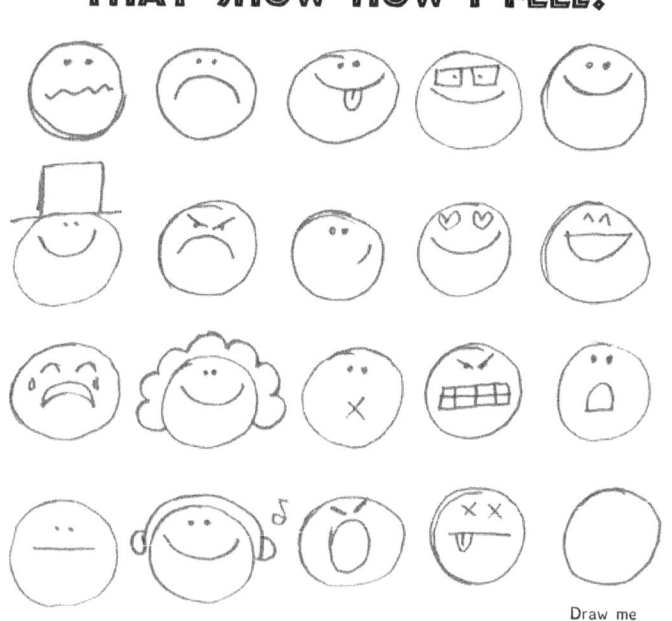

What color are my eyes?

Color my eyes.

Trace my face!
I am using a:
_ Black Pen
_ Colored Pencil
_ Marker
_ Gel Pen
_ Crayon
_ #2 Pencil

Write one word to describe me:

COLOR THE FACES THAT SHOW HOW I FEEL:

Draw me

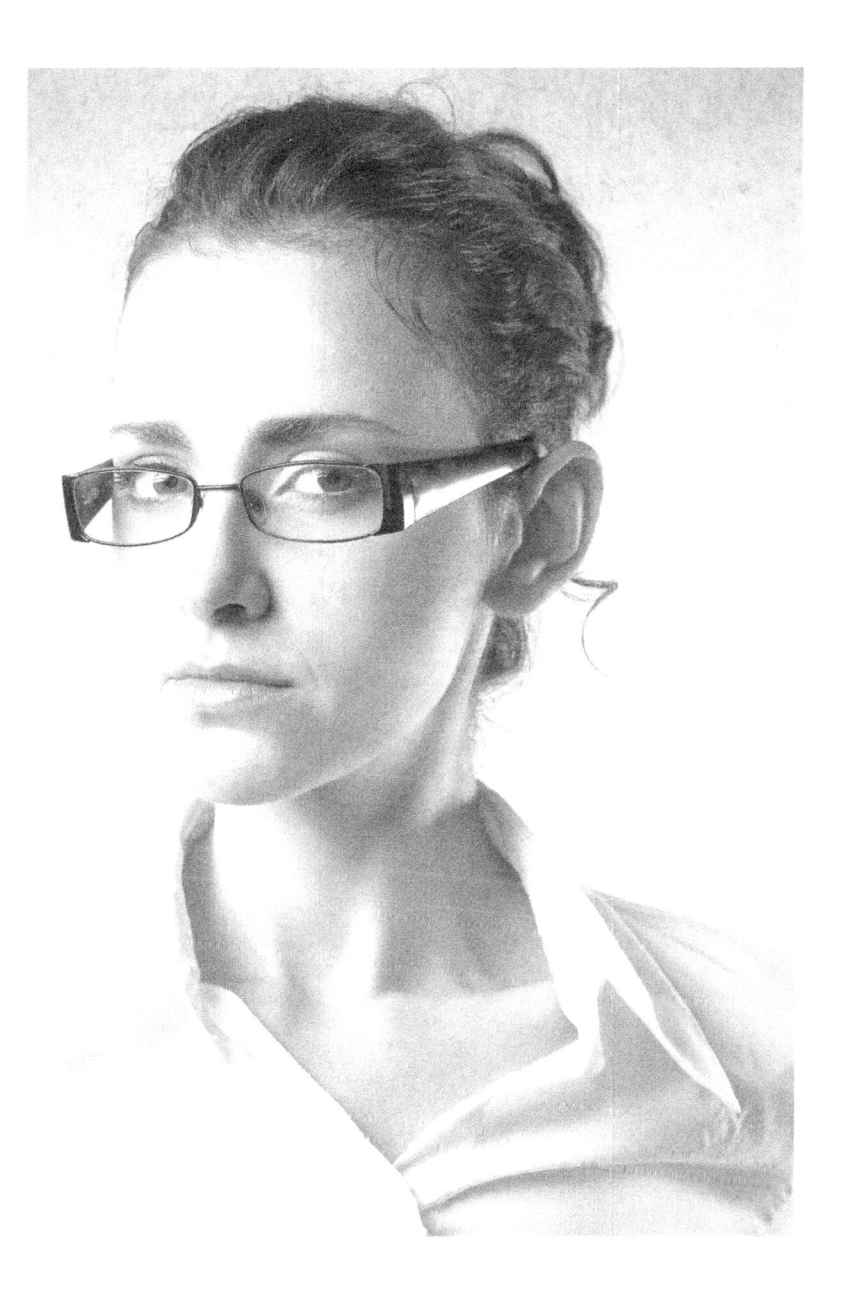

LOOK AT MY FACE!

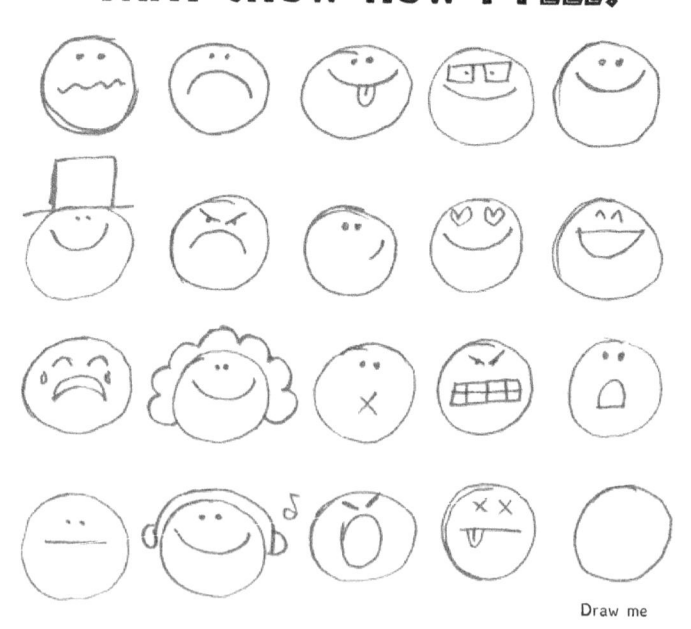

What color are my eyes?

Color my eyes.

Trace my face!
I am using a:
_ Black Pen
_ Colored Pencil
_ Marker
_ Gel Pen
_ Crayon
_ #2 Pencil

Write one word to describe me:

COLOR THE FACES THAT SHOW HOW I FEEL:

Draw me

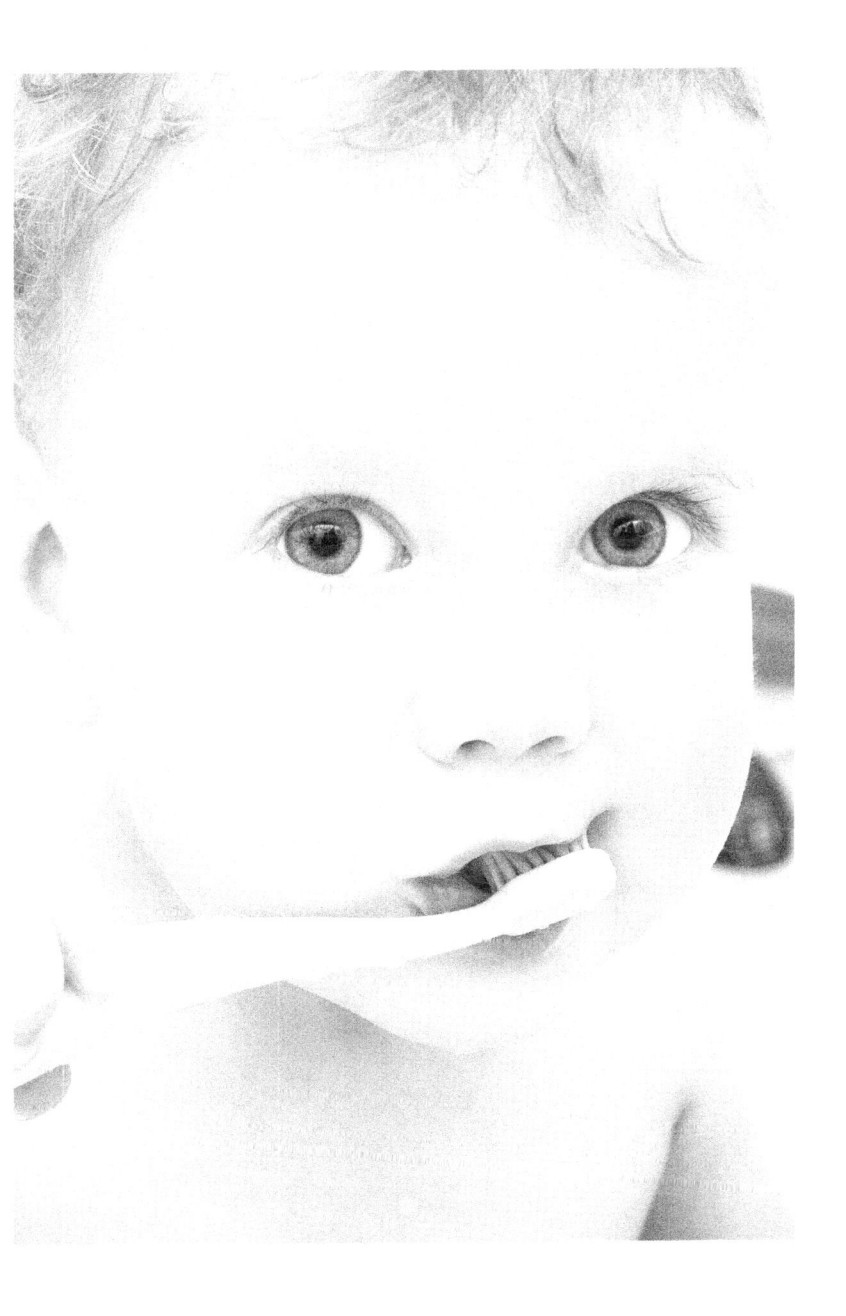

LOOK AT MY FACE!

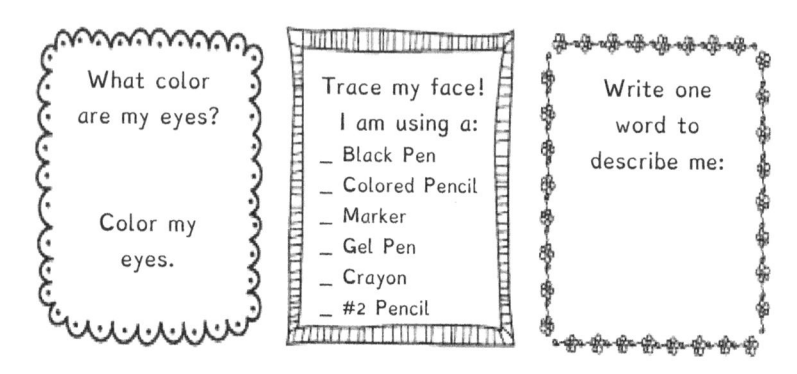

What color are my eyes?

Color my eyes.

Trace my face!
I am using a:
- Black Pen
- Colored Pencil
- Marker
- Gel Pen
- Crayon
- #2 Pencil

Write one word to describe me:

COLOR THE FACES THAT SHOW HOW I FEEL:

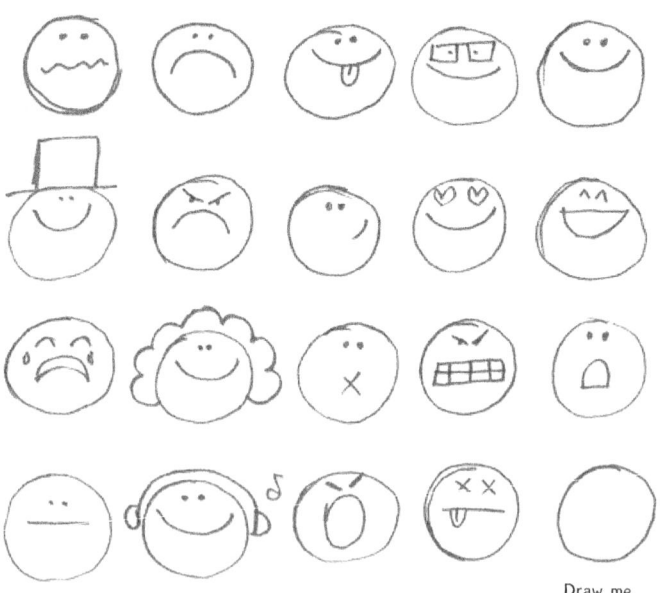

Draw me

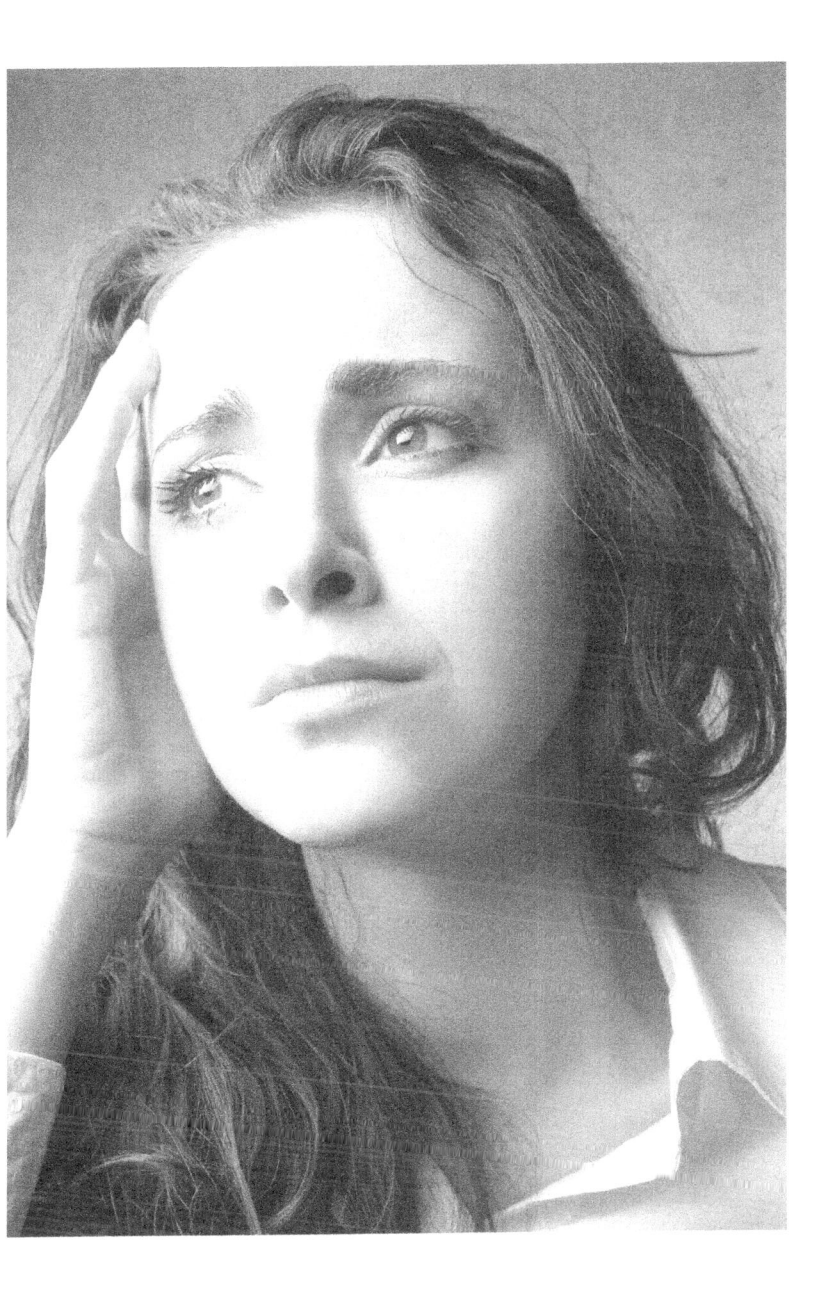

Today I am thinking about:

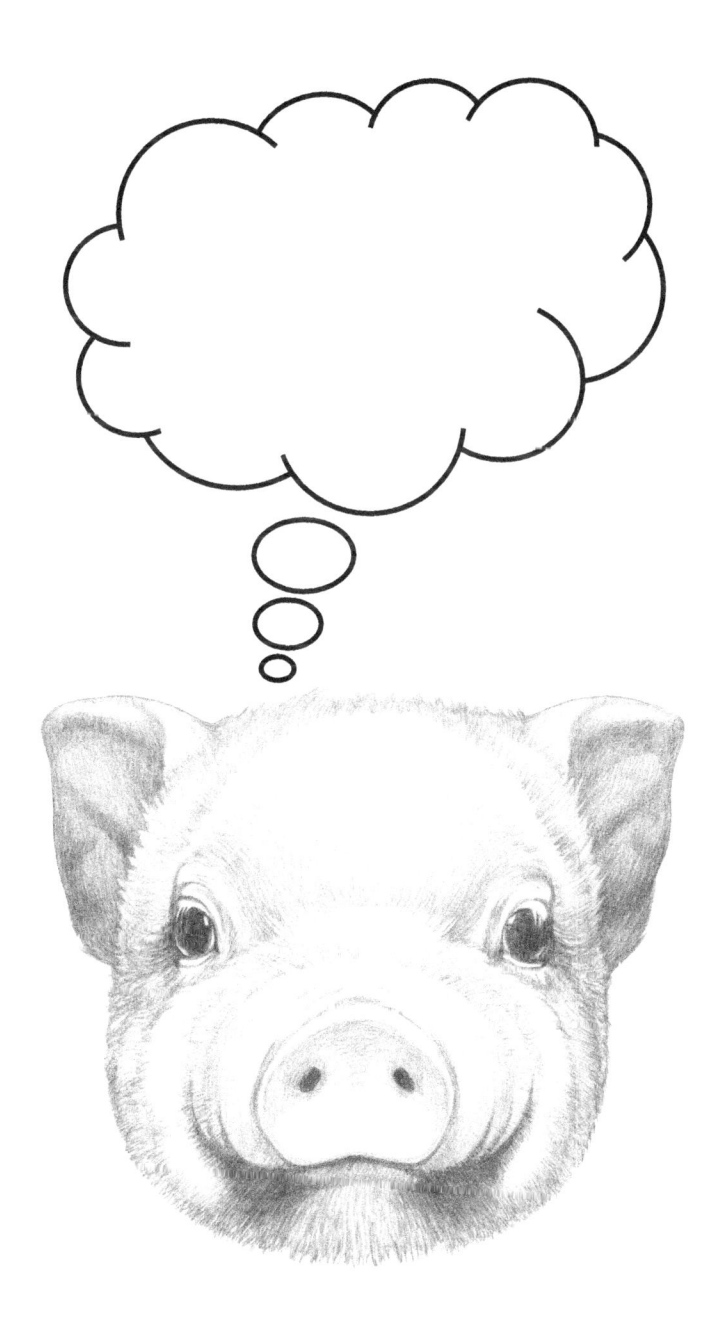

DRAW ANYTHING

LOGIC GAMES

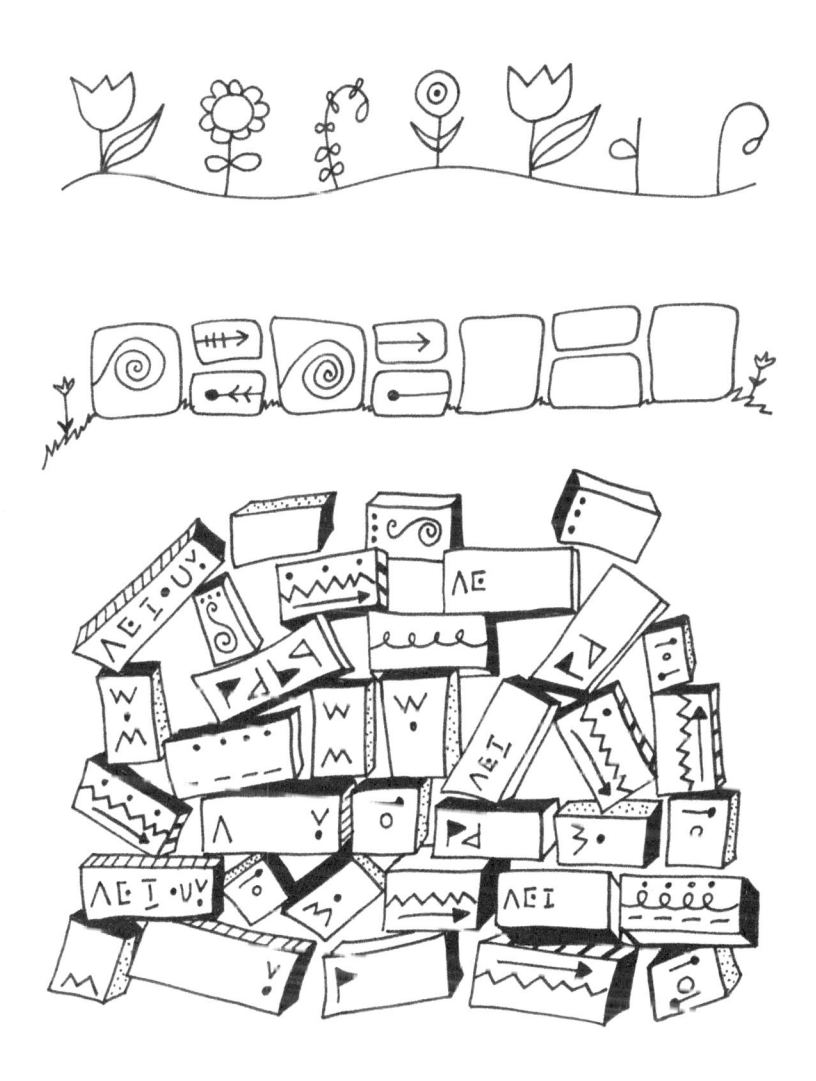

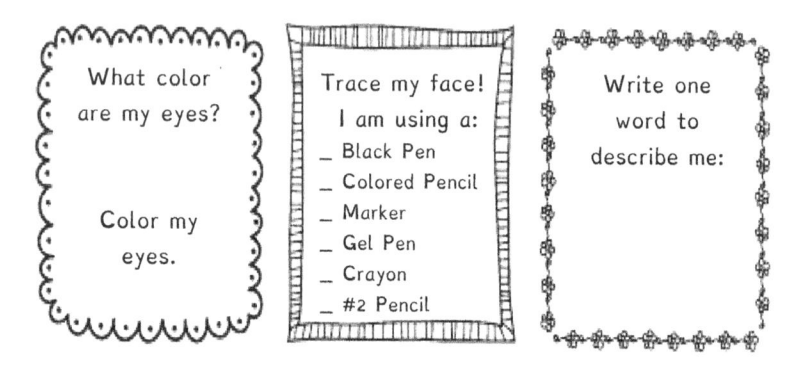

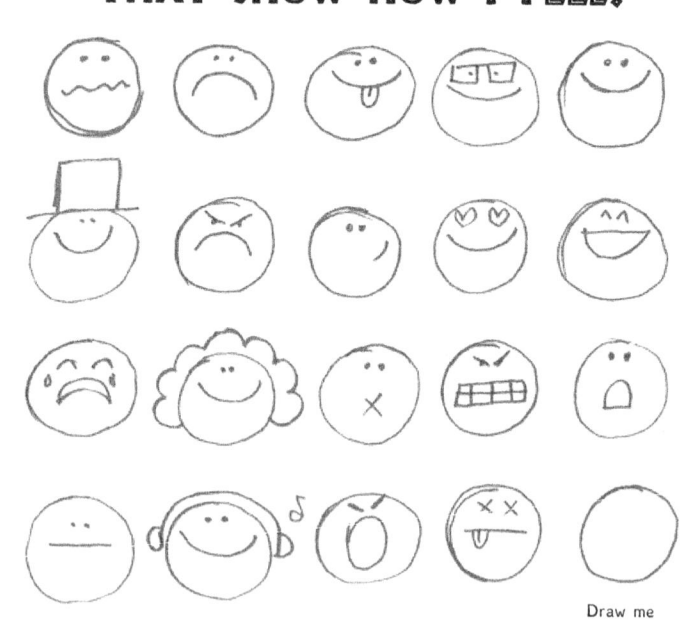

LOOK AT MY FACE!

What color are my eyes?

Color my eyes.

Trace my face!
I am using a:
- _ Black Pen
- _ Colored Pencil
- _ Marker
- _ Gel Pen
- _ Crayon
- _ #2 Pencil

Write one word to describe me:

COLOR THE FACES THAT SHOW HOW I FEEL:

Draw me

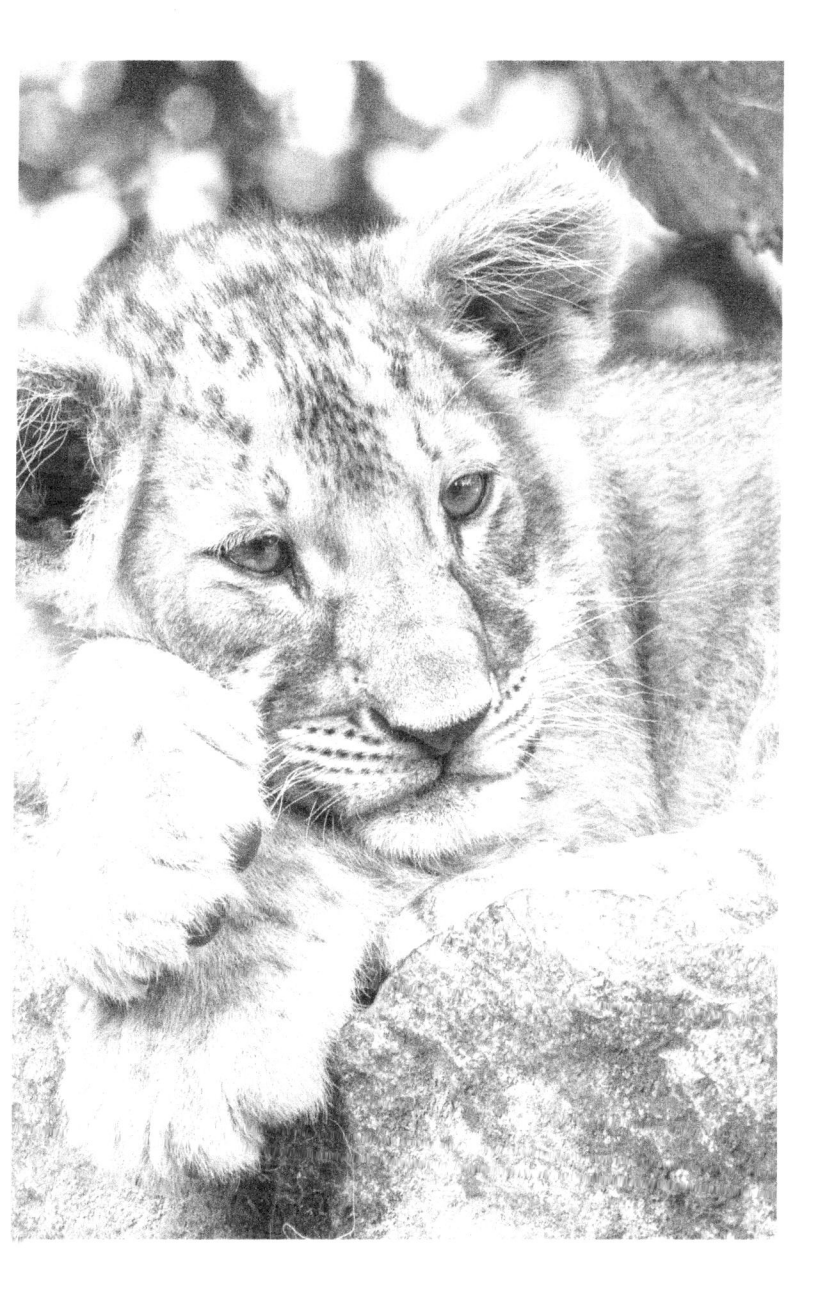

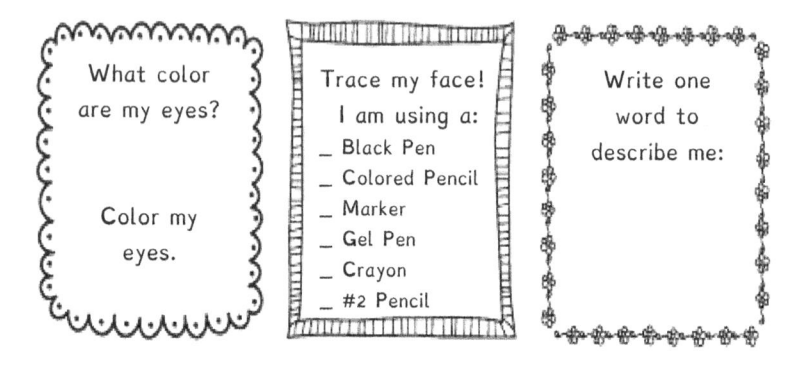

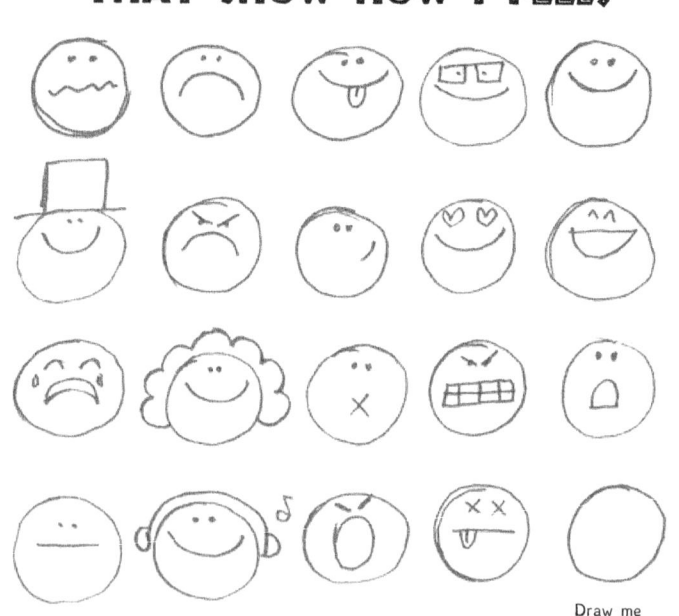

LOOK AT MY FACE!

What color are my eyes?

Color my eyes.

Trace my face!
I am using a:
_ Black Pen
_ Colored Pencil
_ Marker
_ Gel Pen
_ Crayon
_ #2 Pencil

Write one word to describe me:

COLOR THE FACES THAT SHOW HOW I FEEL:

Draw me

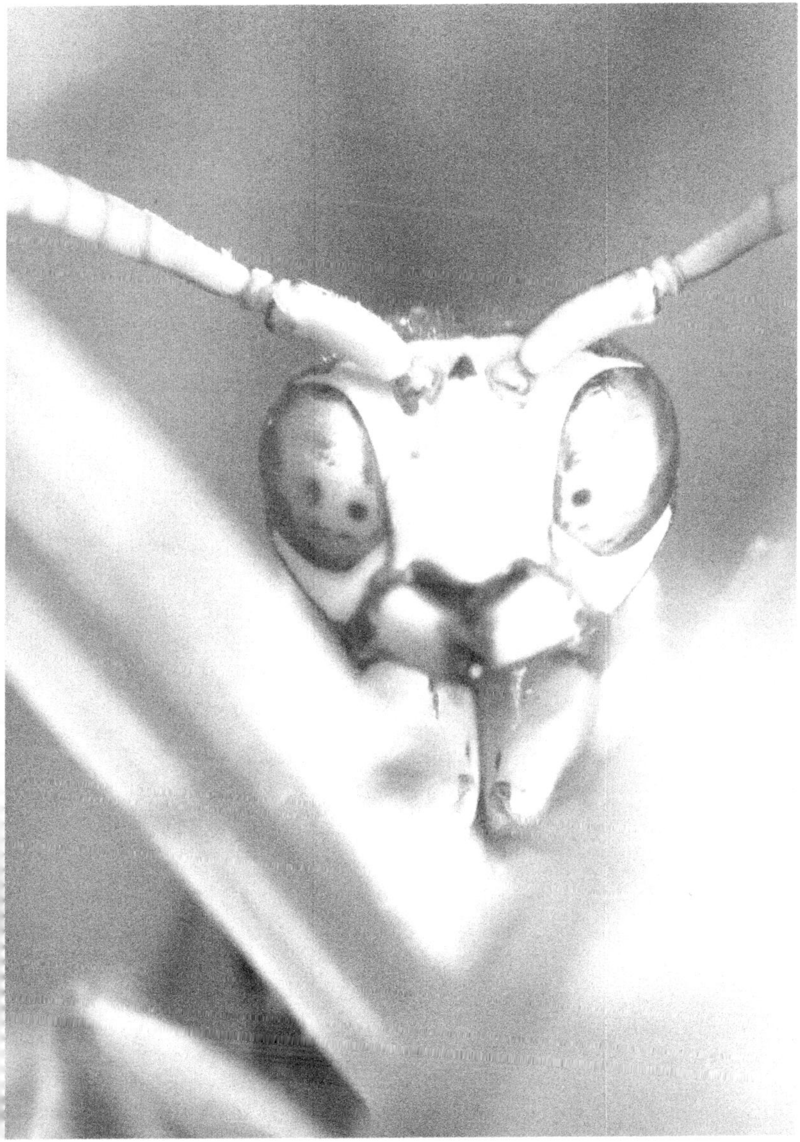

LOOK AT MY FACE!

What color are my eyes?

Color my eyes.

Trace my face!
I am using a:
_ Black Pen
_ Colored Pencil
_ Marker
_ Gel Pen
_ Crayon
_ #2 Pencil

Write one word to describe me:

COLOR THE FACES THAT SHOW HOW I FEEL:

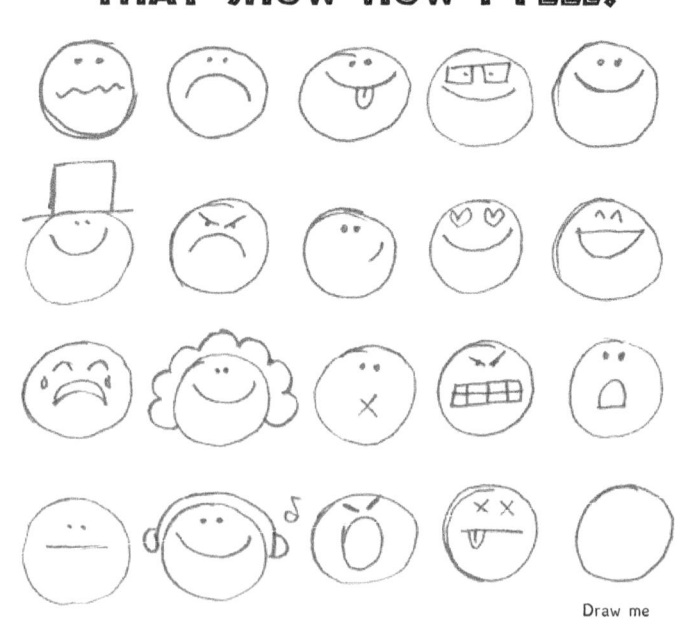

Draw me

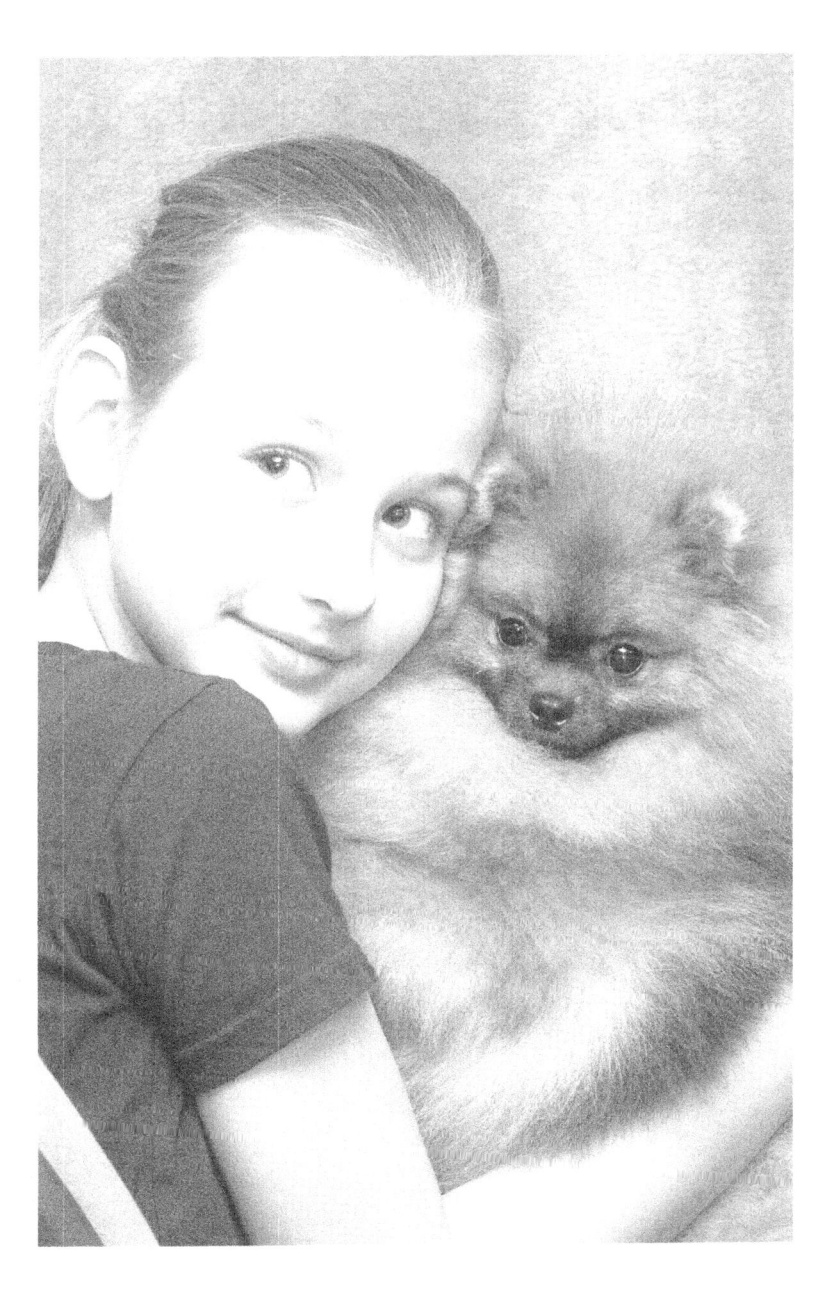

LOOK AT MY FACE!

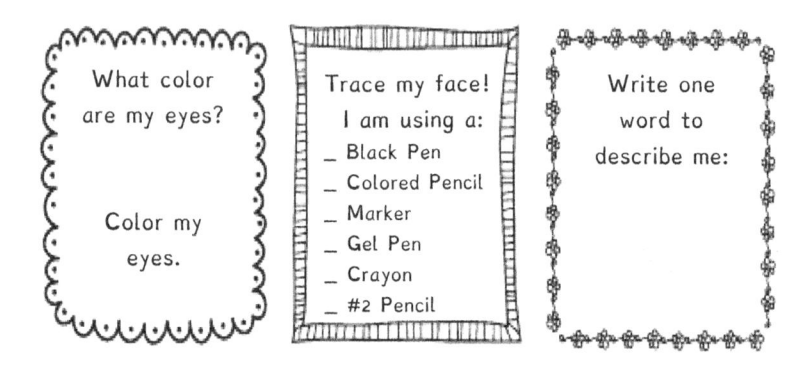

What color are my eyes?

Color my eyes.

Trace my face!
I am using a:
_ Black Pen
_ Colored Pencil
_ Marker
_ Gel Pen
_ Crayon
_ #2 Pencil

Write one word to describe me:

COLOR THE FACES THAT SHOW HOW I FEEL:

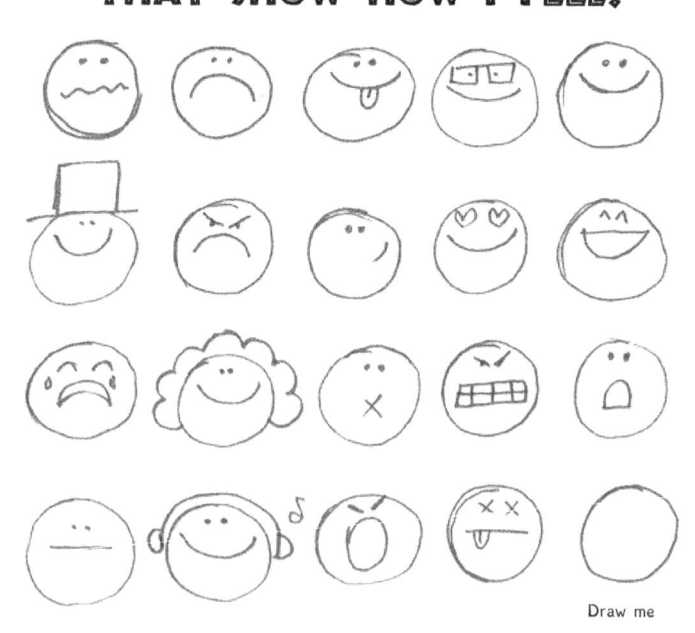

Draw me

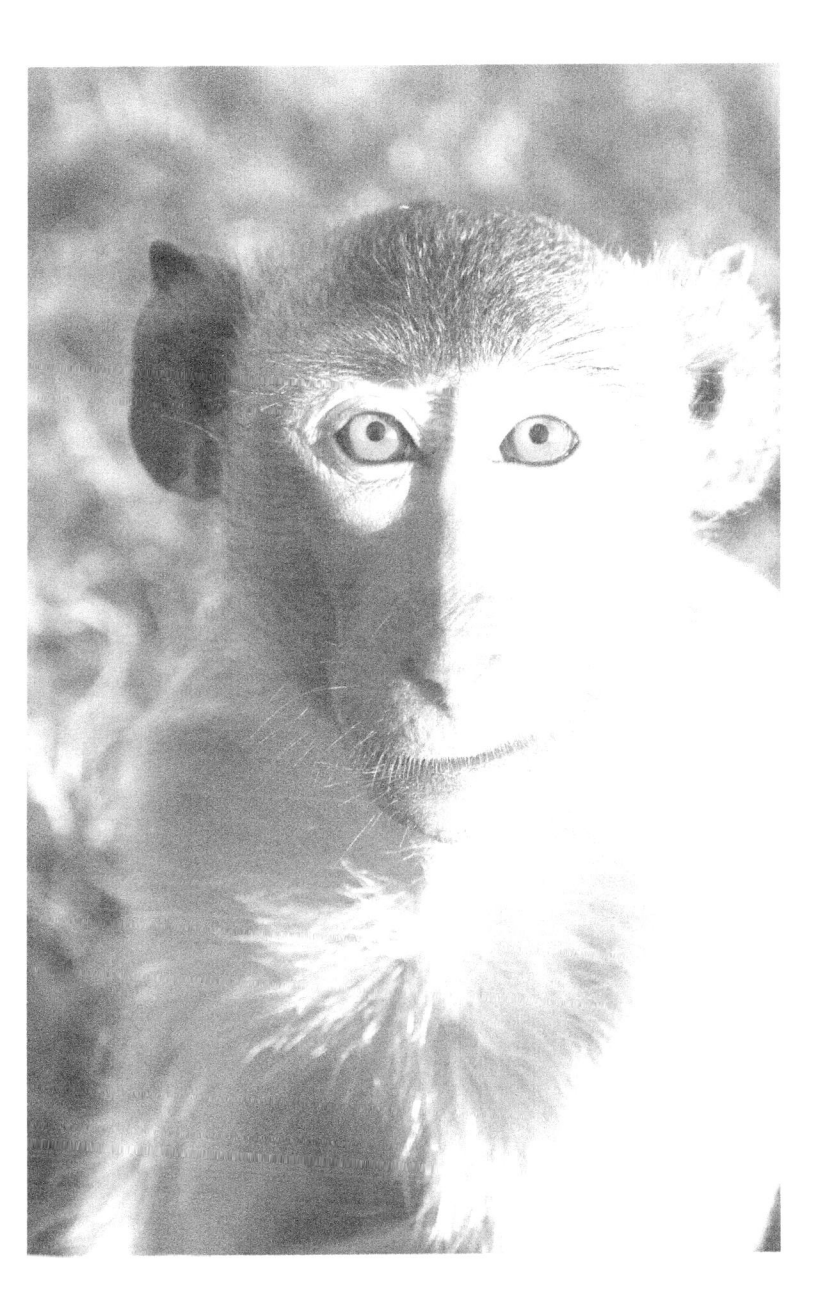

LOOK AT MY FACE!

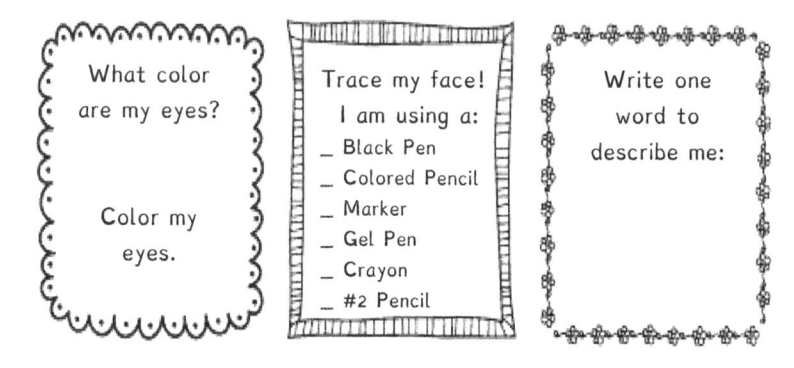

What color are my eyes?

Color my eyes.

Trace my face!
I am using a:
_ Black Pen
_ Colored Pencil
_ Marker
_ Gel Pen
_ Crayon
_ #2 Pencil

Write one word to describe me:

COLOR THE FACES THAT SHOW HOW I FEEL:

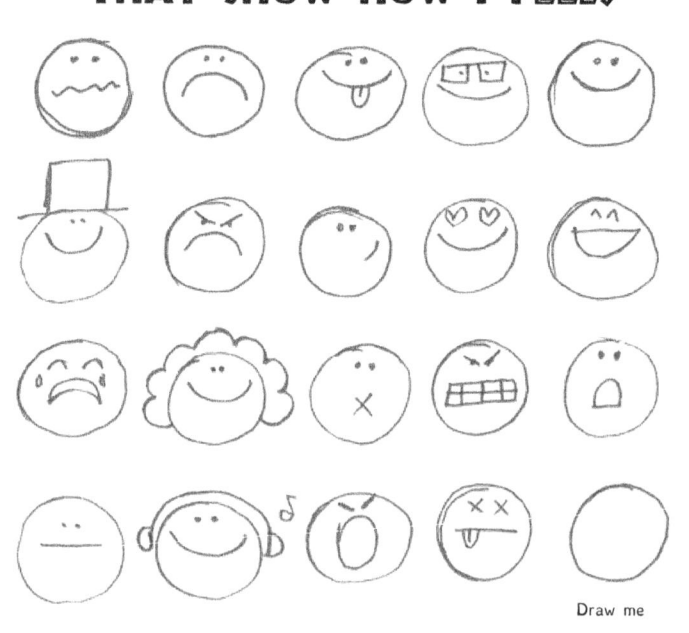

Draw me

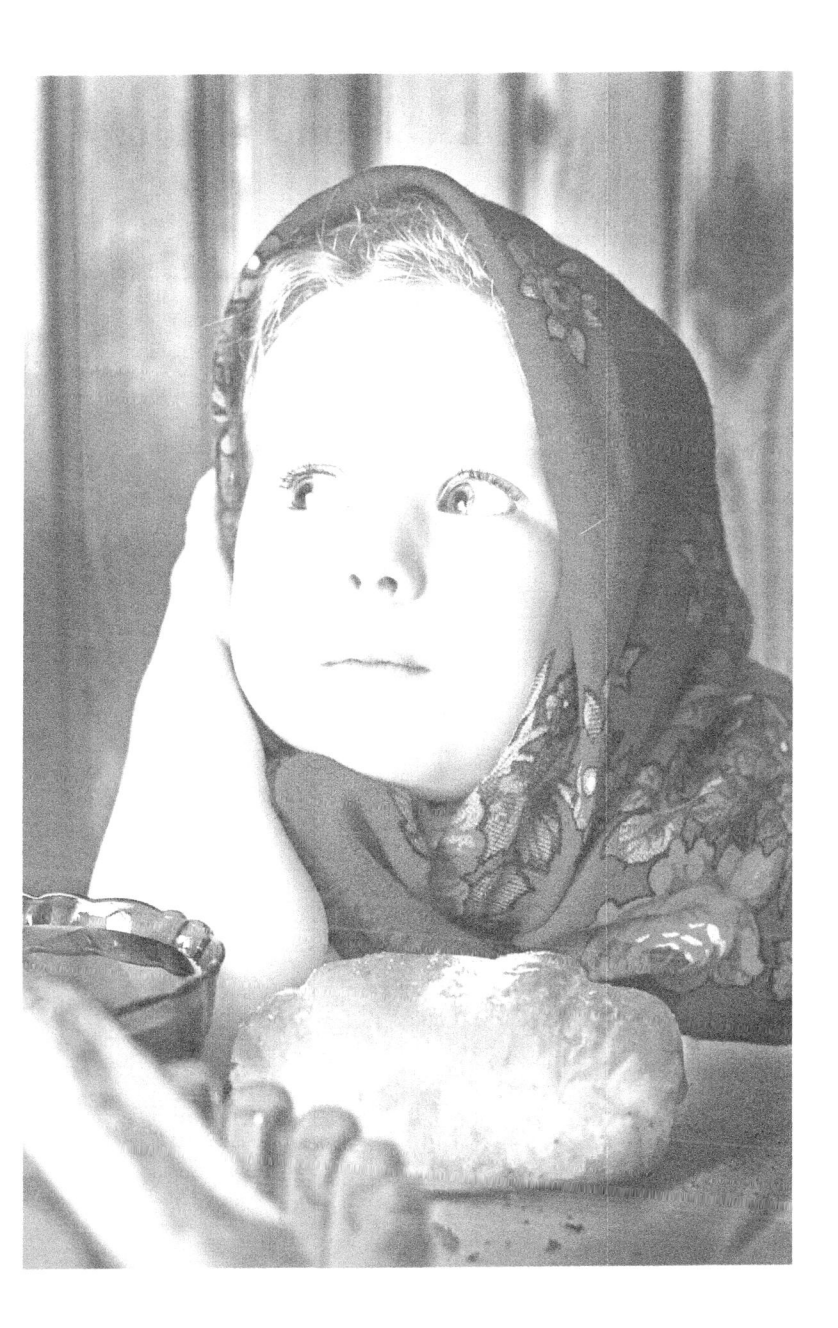

Today I am thinking about:

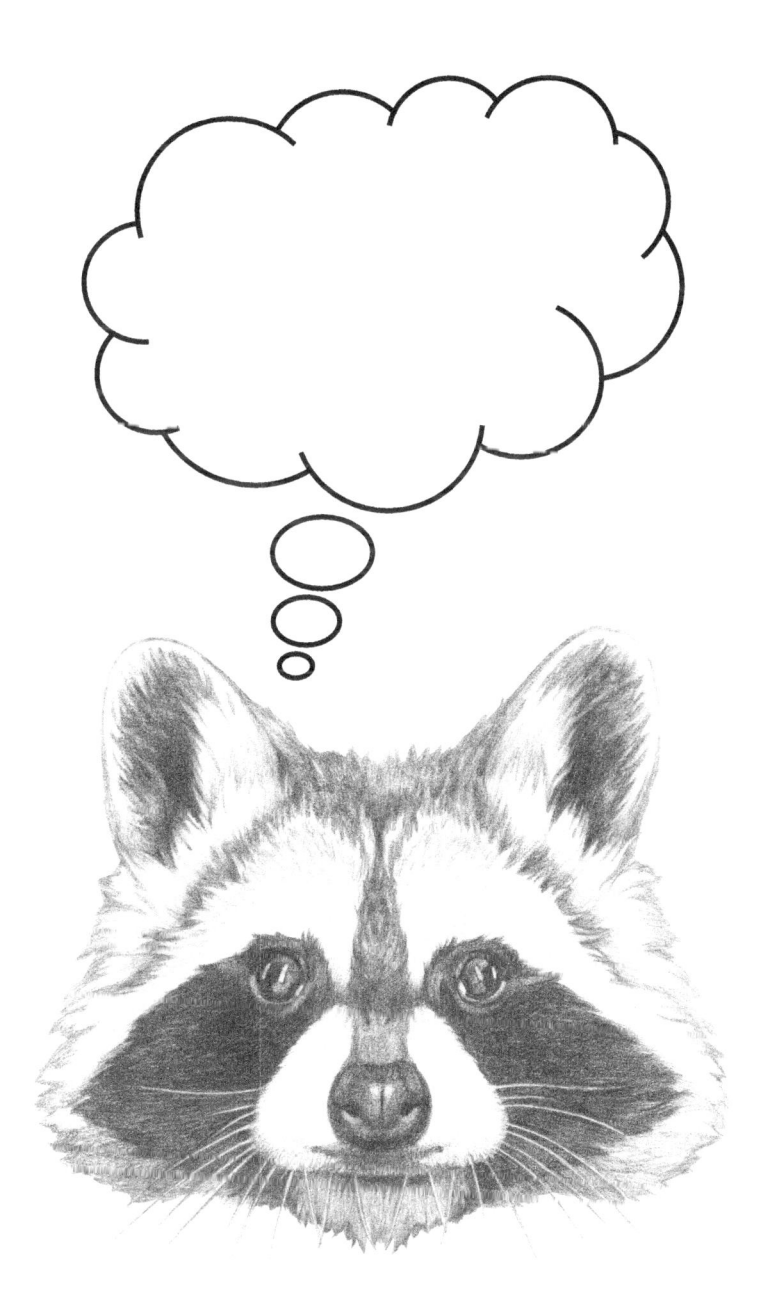

DRAW ANYTHING

LOGIC GAMES

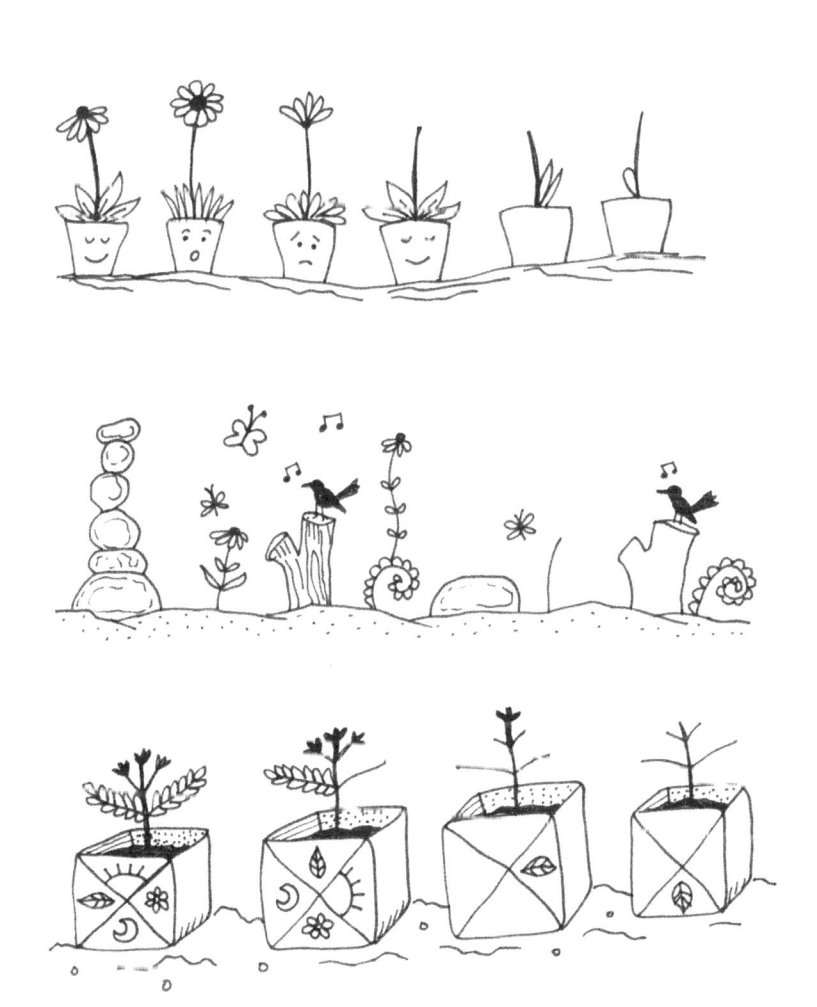

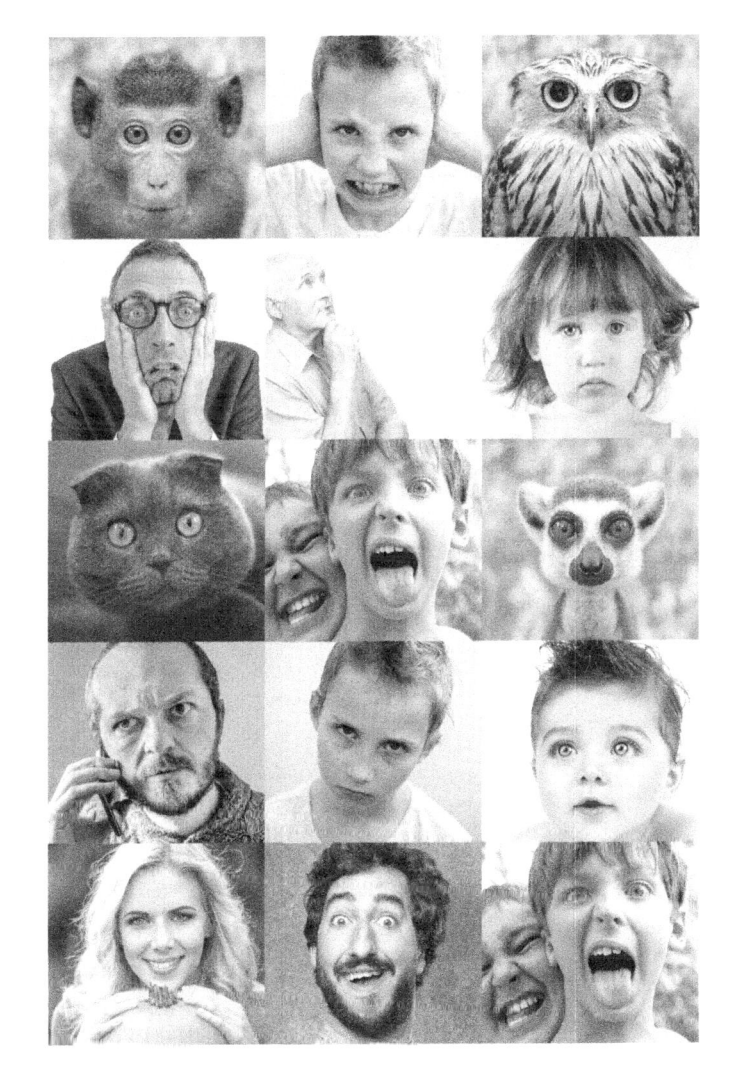

Made in United States
Orlando, FL
12 February 2023